MW00761695

PocketBrain of

CLINICAL
PATHOPHYSIOLOGY

PocketBrain of
CLINICAL
PATHOPHYSIOLOGY

Frank M. Griffin Jr., MD

Senior Vice President
Medical Education and Research
Baptist Health System
Birmingham, Alabama

Professor Emeritus
Department of Medicine
University of Alabama School of Medicine
Birmingham, Alabama

b

**Blackwell
Science**

Blackwell Science

©2001 by Blackwell Science, Inc.

Editorial Offices:
Commerce Place, 350 Main Street, Malden,
Massachusetts 02148, USA
Osney Mead, Oxford OX2 0EL, England
25 John Street, London WC1N 2BL, England
23 Ainslie Place, Edinburgh EH3 6AJ, Scotland
54 University Street, Carlton, Victoria 3053, Australia

Other Editorial Offices:
Blackwell Wissenschafts-Verlag GmbH, Kurfürstendamm 57, 10707 Berlin, Germany
Blackwell Science KK, MG Kodenmacho Building, 7-10 Kodenmacho
    Nihombashi, Chuo-ku, Tokyo 104, Japan
Iowa State University Press, A Blackwell Science Company, 2121 S. State Avenue,
    Ames, Iowa 50014-8300, USA

Distributors:

USA
    Blackwell Science, Inc.
    Commerce Place
    350 Main Street
    Malden, Massachusetts 02148
    (Telephone orders: 800-215-1000
                    or 781-388-8250;
    fax orders: 781-388-8270)

Canada
    Login Brothers Book Company
    324 Saulteaux Crescent
    Winnipeg, Manitoba R3J 3T2
    (Telephone orders: 204-837-2987)

Australia
    Blackwell Science Pty, Ltd.
    54 University Street
    Carlton, Victoria 3053
    (Telephone orders: 03-9347-0300;
    fax orders: 03-9349-3016)

Outside North America and Australia
    Blackwell Science, Ltd.
    c/o Marston Book Services, Ltd.
    P.O. Box 269
    Abingdon
    Oxon OX14 4YN
    England
    (Telephone orders: 44-01235-465500;
    fax orders: 44-01235-465555)

Acquisitions: Beverly Copland
Development: Angela Gagliano
Production: Irene Herlihy
Manufacturing: Lisa Flanagan
Marketing Manager: Toni Fournier
Cover design by Leslie Haimes
Interior design by Gallagher
Typeset by Gallagher
Printed and bound by Sheridan Books

Printed in the United States of America
01 02 03 04 5 4 3 2 1

The Blackwell Science logo is a trade mark of Blackwell Science Ltd.,
registered at the United Kingdom Trade Marks Registry

Library of Congress Cataloging-in-Publication Data
Griffin, Frank M., 1941–
    Pocket brain of clinical pathophysiology / Frank M. Griffin, Jr.
        p. ; cm.
    includes index.
    ISBN 0-632-04634-1 (pbk.)
    1. Physiology, Pathological—Handbooks, manuals, etc.
    [DNLM: 1. Pathology—Handbooks. 2. Diagnostic Techniques and
    Procedures—Handbooks. QZ 39 G851p 2001] I. Title.
    RB113 .G665 2001
    616.07--dc21   2001001142

Contents

Foreword

If one believes that the ability to think will triumph over the ability to remember details, Dr. Griffin's book contains the battle plan for that triumph. It is easy for physicians still in training and those in practice to remember the horror of trying to memorize hundreds of details in the first two years of medical school. Much of what was memorized is retained only for a short time and then forgotten. Suddenly, on arrival to the wards, the medical student is confronted with real patient-care issues that are not even duplicated in case-based basic science courses currently in vogue. The long-forgotten facts from days past easily become humbled in the maze of patient complaints, real physical findings, and preparation for rounds.

During my own training, I was fortunate to work extensively with Dr. Griffin. Over the course of my training and career, his teaching has helped me to reason through many complicated patient problems by using logic along with a few basic facts and principles of pathophysiology that are outlined in this excellent book. Many alumni of his rotations have hoped he would publish just such a book as this.

Regardless of your level of training, from medical student to attending physician, I am confident you will find Dr. Griffin's approach to be interesting, surprisingly simple, and intellectually stimulating. I also believe that you will find that this book will alter your approach to problems not addressed herein, by teaching you to think about mechanisms of disease rather than relying on memory alone.

Enjoy the solution to the maze.

Gorman R. Jones, MD
Director of Medical Clinics
Internal Medicine Residency Program
Baptist Health Systems
Birmingham, Alabama

Preface

Practicing medicine is a great source of enjoyment for me in two very important ways: the pleasure of interpersonal relationships with patients and colleagues, and the intellectual joy of figuring out complex problems. Solving complicated clinical problems is accomplished most efficiently by reasoning pathophysiologically—that is, by trying to understand a patient's complaints and problems in terms of the underlying pathophysiologic mechanisms that explain them. Once we understand the physiologic basis for a clinical problem, then differential diagnoses follow automatically.

Over the years I have attended on internal medicine services, I noticed that many of the same clinical problems arose month after month. Students and house officers had varying degrees of understanding of these problems, and even those who had the greatest knowledge about them often did not understand the underlying pathophysiology thoroughly. This book is intended to provide a framework for understanding the pathophysiologic basis of several commonly encountered clinical problems and the pathophysiologic reasoning used in solving them. Pathophysiologic reasoning is very powerful. It allows physicians to make a diagnosis of a disease that they did not know existed; I have seen students and house officers do just that many times in my career. I have recorded several of these spectacular moments in the clinical vignettes included throughout this book.

I have tried to keep things simple and to provide a basic understanding of mechanisms, not necessarily to provide a complete differential diagnosis of every problem. More complete discussions can be found in many excellent textbooks.

As the title suggests, this book is intended to be used as a "pocket brain" to help students, house officers, and other interested physicians reason pathophysiologically through clinical problems. I hope readers will have as much fun using the book as I did writing it.

Acknowledgments

I am deeply indebted to my mentors and colleagues and am especially grateful to the students, residents, and fellows who have taught me so much and made medicine so much fun for more than 30 years. I thank Valerie Webster and Margaret Williams for preparing the manuscript.

FMG

Notice

The indications and dosages of all drugs in this book have been recommended in the medical literature and conform to the practices of the general community. The medications described and treatment prescriptions suggested do not necessarily have specific approval by the Food and Drug Administration for use in the diseases and dosages for which they are recommended. The package insert for each drug should be consulted for use and dosage as approved by the FDA. Because standards for usage change, it is advisable to keep abreast of revised recommendations, particularly those concerning new drugs.

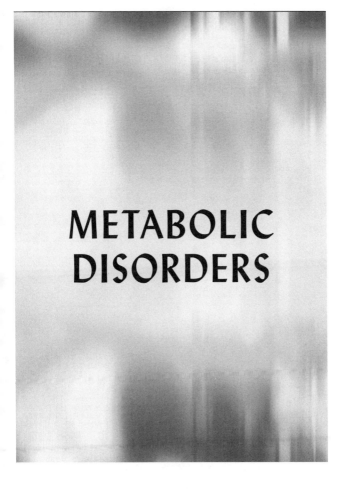

PART

I

METABOLIC DISORDERS

1

Hyponatremia

There are only two mechanisms by which one can become hyponatremic: by overwhelming the kidney's ability to dilute urine and by elaborating the molecule antidiuretic hormone (ADH). In a patient with hyponatremia, determining the osmolality of the urine will readily distinguish between these two mechanisms. When the kidney's ability to dilute urine has been overwhelmed, the urine osmolality will be low, generally less than 100 mOsm/L. When ADH is responsible, the urine osmolality will be higher, almost always greater than 300 mOsm/L (Figure 1.1).

Hyponatremia as a result of the kidney's ability to dilute urine being overwhelmed is very rare. People with normal renal function can drink 20 liters or more of water a day without becoming hyponatremic, because the normal kidney is able to excrete that much or more. Even patients with severely impaired renal function—for example, those whose renal function is only 10% of normal—are nevertheless able to excrete at least 2 to 3 liters of free water per day. Thus, one encounters hyponatremia due to this mechanism only in psychiatrically ill patients who imbibe huge quantities of water. As indicated in Figure 1.1, this mechanism is easily proven or excluded by the simple determination of urine osmolality in a hyponatremic patient.

Thus, essentially all hyponatremia is mediated by ADH. Under physiologic conditions and under many pathologic conditions, the level of ADH regulates and is regulated by

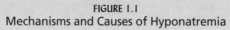

FIGURE 1.1
Mechanisms and Causes of Hyponatremia

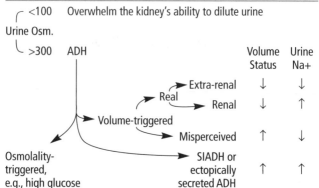

serum osmolality. Thus, when serum osmolality is high, as in a patient with severe hyperglycemia, ADH will be released in higher quantities and will result in increased absorption of free water, thereby diluting all components of the blood, including sodium. In addition, the increased osmolality of the extracellular compartment will cause water to shift from the intracellular compartment, thereby further diluting serum components. Hyponatremia caused by hyperglycemia is never a mystery because as soon as physicians know a patient is hyponatremic, they also know the patient is hyperglycemic because both sodium and glucose determinations appear on a chemistry seven profile.

Thus, two primary causes of hyponatremia, compulsive water drinking and hyperosmolality due to hyperglycemia, are readily provable or are immediately obvious to the physician and should never prove difficult to prove or to diagnose. Likewise, pseudohyponatremia of hyperlipidemic serum is not a difficult diagnostic problem. Here, sodium is contained in the water space of serum but is reported over the entire volume of serum including lipid; thus, the patient is not physiologically hyponatremic. Pseudohyponatremia should not be a diagnostic problem for the physician because the laboratory personnel should note that the serum is hyperlipemic.

All hyponatremia that is diagnostically difficult is mediated by ADH. ADH may be either secreted inappropriately or elaborated by a neoplastic cell, or it may be elaborated in response to volume depletion that may be real or may be misperceived by volume sensors. We must distinguish among four physiologic states to identify the cause of hyponatremia once the three causes discussed in earlier paragraphs are excluded. We can do this by obtaining two determinations: first, estimate the patient's volume status by clinical examination; second, measure the urine sodium concentration (see Figure 1.1). Volume depletion sensed by volume receptors may be either real or misperceived. If real, volume depletion may have occurred by renal or by extrarenal fluid losses. Finally, hyponatremia may be caused by either the syndrome of inappropriate secretion of ADH (SIADH) or secretion of ADH by a neoplastic cell.

In volume depletion that results from extrarenal fluid losses, the patient will appear volume-depleted clinically, and the urine sodium will be very low because of aldosterone and other sodium-conserving renal mechanisms. In volume depletion that is due to renal losses of fluid, such as in Addison's disease, the patient will clinically appear volume-depleted but the urine sodium will be elevated. The most common cause of misperceived volume depletion is cardiac dysfunction that results in such poor cardiac output that volume receptors misperceive a hypovolemic state. Here, as in the two physiologic conditions just discussed, ADH is elaborated in response to perceived volume depletion, even though causing the absorption of free water in a patient who has iso-osmolar serum will make the patient hypo-osmolar. A less common cause of hyponatremia caused by misperceived volume depletion occurs in severe hepatic disease, often in the presence of impending or actual hepatorenal syndrome. In both cardiac failure and liver failure the patient will be clinically hypervolemic and the urine sodium will be very low, again because of aldosterone and other sodium-conserving renal mechanisms.

Finally, patients with either ectopic secretion of ADH or SIADH will appear either euvolemic or slightly hyper-volemic. The urine sodium will be very high because aldos-terone and other renal salt-conserving mechanisms will be downregulated due to hypervolemia.

As seen in Figure 1.1, the physiologic cause of a patient's hyponatremia should become readily apparent, assuming that the physician accurately assesses the patient's volume status and that there are no problems such as recent diuretic administration to confound the interpreta-tion of the urine sodium.

To review, the logical sequence for approaching a patient with hyponatremia is as follows:

1. Be certain that the serum is not hyperlipemic.
2. Determine the urine osmolality to distinguish between the two mechanisms by which hyponatremia can occur (i.e., overwhelming the kidney's ability to dilute urine, and ADH).
3. Be certain that the serum is not hyperosmolar, usually due to marked hyperglycemia.
4. Determine the patient's volume status clinically and the urine sodium concentration to identify which of the four pathophysiologic causes (see Figure 1.1) best explains the patient's hyponatremia.

CLINICAL VIGNETTE

A 35-year-old man presented with progressively severe weakness and easy fatigability of several months' dura-tion. His blood pressure was 105/55, and his heart rate increased from 90 to 115 on standing. The laboratory evaluation revealed that he had a mild lymphocytosis and 10% eosinophilia. His serum sodium level was 125 mEq/L, potassium was 5.6 mEq/L, bicarbonate was 14 mEq/L, and glucose was 55 mg/dL. (The patient has hyponatremia, hyperkalemia, metabolic acidosis, hypoglycemia, low serum osmolality, and eosinophilia, all of which will be discussed in subsequent chapters. The current focus is on hyponatremia.)

When evaluating the patient's hyponatremia, the house-staff first checked with the laboratory to be sure that his serum was not hyperlipemic. They measured his urine osmolality and found it to be 350 mOsm/L, indicating that the mechanism of hyponatremia was excessive ADH. They noted that his serum glucose was not elevated, and they calculated his serum osmolality and determined that it was not elevated but low.

After excluding the above causes of hyponatremia, they then assessed his volume status and measured the level of his urine sodium. Because the patient's blood pressure was low and his heart rate increased on standing, they judged his volume status to be low. His urine sodium level was 85 mEq/L. The house-staff concluded that the patient was truly volume depleted and that volume depletion was a consequence of a salt-wasting nephropathy. The clinical features of his illness, his laboratory data, and the house-staff's evaluation for the cause of hyponatremia all suggested that the patient had adrenal insufficiency. Measurement of his serum cortisol before and after administration of Cortrosyn revealed all levels to be under 5 µg/dL. The house-staff concluded that the patient had adrenal insufficiency, treated him with cortisol, and set out to determine whether his adrenal insufficiency was primary or secondary.

Even though the diagnosis of adrenal insufficiency was strongly suggested by all of the features with which the patient presented, the house-staff nevertheless went through the proper logical sequence to prove the mechanism for his hyponatremia. When they found that the patient had a salt-wasting nephropathy, they proved the suspected diagnosis by measuring the serum cortisol levels.

2

Hypernatremia

Hypernatremia occurs in situations in which water is lost and not replaced. Because all volume losses—whether they be from the gastrointestinal tract, kidney, skin, or lungs—are hyponatremic relative to plasma, hypernatremia will always result if water is not adequately replaced. Hypernatremia is encountered in two fundamental situations: in patients with diabetes insipidus, and in patients who lose volume and free water from extrarenal sources and are unable to drink. The latter are usually helpless individuals who are unable to gain access to water; often they are demented. The two fundamental causes can be readily distinguished by simply determining the urine osmolality or specific gravity. In diabetes insipidus they will be low; in other conditions of hypernatremia they will be high. Salt water near-drowning, a third cause of hypernatremia, is generally diagnostically obvious and I will not discuss it further.

Patients with diabetes insipidus often have a nearly pure free water deficit, and their hypernatremia can be corrected by administering free water (D5W). In contrast, patients with hypernatremia not caused by diabetes insipidus are always volume depleted, usually markedly so, and fluid therapy should be directed toward correcting the volume deficit first. Therefore, treatment should begin with normal saline. Note that saline, which contains 154 mEq/L of sodium, is actually hypotonic to the serum of patients with significant hypernatremia. Therefore, even when patients receive saline, hypernatremia will be partially corrected.

One can calculate a patient's free water deficit by knowing the patient's weight and the normal amount of water in the body (60% of the body is water), and by multiplying the patient's body water weight by the fraction above eunatremic the patient's serum is. For example, if we use 140 mEq/L as normal serum sodium, a 70-kg patient whose serum sodium is 168 mEq/L would have a 20% free water deficit of 8.4 liters; we calculate this by multiplying his weight (70 kg) by 0.6 (the fraction of his body that is water), and multiplying the result by 28/140, which is his serum sodium's fraction above normal. Although it is useful to understand how that formula is derived, I find it not very important in managing hypernatremic patients. The goals of treatment should be first to substantially or completely correct the volume deficit and then to complete the correction of the water deficit over approximately 2 days. This can be accomplished either by completely correcting the volume deficit with saline and then switching to D5W, or by partially correcting the volume deficit and then switching to half normal saline and only later to D5W.

3

Metabolic Acidosis

Metabolic acidosis may be of the anion gap or non-gap type. The non-gap metabolic acidoses include the various forms of renal tubular acidosis, loss of bicarbonate from the gastrointestinal tract because of diarrhea, and loss of bicarbonate and reabsorption of chloride when urine is allowed to stand in an ileal conduit. In the last instance, obstruction of the ileal conduit allows urine to remain in the conduit for prolonged periods. The ileum acts on the pooled urine as it normally does with gastrointestinal contents: it reabsorbs chloride and excretes bicarbonate. The presence of hyperchloremic metabolic acidosis in a patient with an ileal conduit should lead the physician to investigate the possibility that there is a mechanical defect leading to obstruction of urine flow through the conduit.

Metabolic acidosis associated with an anion gap may be due to accumulation of endogenous acid or the introduction of exogenous acid. There are only three endogenous causes of metabolic acidosis associated with an anion gap: ketosis, lactic acidosis, and renal failure resulting in the accumulation of phosphates and sulfates. Exogenous causes are similarly few, and include the ingestion of methanol (which is converted to formic acid), ethylene glycol, paraldehyde, or large quantities of salicylates.

Acidosis due to renal failure is usually immediately obvious from the determination of the blood urea nitrogen (BUN) and creatinine levels. Diabetic ketoacidosis is likewise usually obvious; the glucose is generally quite high and ketones are present in high titer in the blood. The more difficult diagnostic problems include distinguishing among lactic acidosis, acidosis due to ingestion of an exogenous acid, and ketoacidosis that is not due to diabetes. When ingestion of exogenous acid is suspected, one should measure the serum osmolality and determine whether there is a substantial difference between the osmolality measured and that which is calculated in the standard fashion (see Chapter 8). If there is a gap, one should measure the blood salicylate level, examine the urine carefully looking for the crystals characteristic of ethylene glycol ingestion, and seek evidence for ingestion of methanol. It is critically important to identify the particular acid that was ingested, because each acid has a very specific treatment.

When there is no evidence of ingestion of an exogenous acid and when the patient is not in diabetic ketoacidosis and does not have renal failure, the major differential diagnostic considerations are lactic acidosis and ketoacidosis due either to starvation or to alcoholism. These can usually be readily distinguished by determining the blood levels of the specific acids. However, alcoholic ketoacidosis is characterized by fairly low levels of acetoacetate and acetone and very high levels of β-hydroxybutyrate, which is not detected by the standard measurement of ketone bodies. Thus, this diagnosis is made by the clinical setting and by excluding other causes.

CLINICAL VIGNETTE

A 20-year-old woman was brought to the emergency room because of dyspnea and confusion. The patient had noted the onset of dyspnea about 12 hours prior to her hospital admission, and it had become progressively severe since then. Her friends had noted her progressive confusion for about an hour. On physical examination she was confused, her respiratory rate was 25, and her breaths were noted to be long and deep. The remainder of the physical examination including the examination of the lungs was unremarkable. Her chest radiograph was normal. The laboratory evaluation revealed a serum glucose level of 15 mg/dL, bicarbonate of 5 mEq/L, and an arterial pH of 7.0. Her urine revealed no ketones, her renal function was normal, and her serum lactate level was normal.

The house-staff realized at this point that all endogenous causes of anion gap metabolic acidosis had been excluded. They obtained a salicylate level that was negative, and they measured her serum osmolality. The serum osmolality by measurement was 340 mOsm/L; however, the calculated serum osmolality was only 275 mOsm/L, thus indicating the presence of an unmeasured, osmotically active molecule. The house-staff felt that the combination of severe anion gap metabolic acidosis and hypoglycemia was most consistent with the ingestion of methanol. They immediately began treating the patient with an ethanol infusion. After more insistent questioning of the patient's friends, the house-staff learned that the patient and her friends had had a party the night before at which the patient had consumed fairly large quantities of wood alcohol.

Because the patient was treated promptly for methanol ingestion, she suffered no optic nerve damage and her dyspnea, acidosis, and hypoglycemia resolved progressively over the ensuing 24 hours.

4

Lactic Acidosis

Lactate is generated by anaerobic glycolysis. It is normally converted to pyruvate and metabolized by the liver via the Krebs cycle. Understanding these principles leads to the differential diagnosis of lactic acidosis. The most common cause of lactic acidosis, and one which we all experience frequently, is generating more lactic acid by exercise than can be immediately metabolized. When we exert ourselves heavily, we drop our pH to the range of 7.0 because of lactate accumulation. That profound acidosis is the reason we are so dyspneic with exercise. As we rest, the lactate is converted to pyruvate, which is rapidly metabolized. The most common pathologic cause of lactic acidosis is hypoperfusion of tissues so that oxygen in not available to metabolize lactate via the Krebs cycle. A second pathologic cause is depletion of NAD$^+$ by alcohol, which impairs the conversion of lactate to pyruvate. A third pathologic cause is a defect in mitochondria such that lactate cannot be metabolized. Examples include genetic disorders in which an important mitochondrial enzyme is missing or defective, mitochondrial poisoning by metformin and by nucleoside analogs used to treat HIV infection, and cyanide poisoning. Finally, acute but usually not chronic liver failure may result in lactic acidosis because of the liver's inability to metabolize the acid.

CLINICAL VIGNETTE

A woman with HIV infection who was receiving two nucleoside analog drugs was hospitalized after several weeks of protracted nausea and vomiting. Her viral load was very low and her CD4 count 800/μL. The physical examination was unremarkable except for hyperpnea and signs of volume depletion. Her chemistry profile revealed a bicarbonate level of 10 mEq/L with an anion gap of 22 mEq/L. The salicylate level was 0. There was no substantial difference between her measured and calculated serum osmolality. She did not have renal failure, and the serum ketones were negative.

The house-staff reasoned that they had excluded all endogenous and exogenous causes of metabolic acidosis other than lactate. Even though they knew of no reason why she should have lactic acidosis, they measured her blood level of lactate and found it to be 10 mEq/L. A literature search revealed that nucleoside analogs had been previously found to cause lactic acidosis by impairing hepatic mitochondria, thereby rendering them unable to metabolize lactate. The house-staff halted her nucleoside analog treatment, began the administration of intravenous bicarbonate, and consulted with the liver transplant team.

This is an excellent example of the house-staff using very careful and thorough pathophysiologic reasoning to arrive at a diagnosis of a disease they did not know existed.

5

Renal Tubular Acidoses

There are four renal tubular acidoses (RTAs). The cause of Type II RTA is inability of the proximal tubule to absorb bicarbonate. Fanconi's syndrome, a related disorder, is essentially Type II RTA with additional tubular lesions that result in defects in handling other small molecules. In Type II RTA and in Fanconi's syndrome, bicarbonate is lost from the proximal tubule; this results in a large load of sodium bicarbonate delivered to the distal tubule, where because of the large sodium load and under the influence of aldosterone, large quantities of sodium are reabsorbed in exchange for potassium and hydrogen. Thus, the patient will tend to be hypokalemic. In addition, because there is no impairment of hydrogen ion secretion in these disorders, urine pH may be quite acidic, 5.0 or lower. Nevertheless, the large volume of bicarbonate loss results in persistent hyperchloremic metabolic acidosis.

Distal, or Type I, RTA is a defect in the secretion of hydrogen ion. In the distal tubule, sodium will then exchange preferentially for potassium, resulting in a tendency toward hypokalemia. Type IV RTA is real or functional aldosterone deficiency. The lesion may be either diminished production of renin, diminished production of aldosterone, or more commonly end organ insensitivity to aldosterone. Here, there is a defect in the secretion by the distal tubule of both hydrogen and potassium ions, with a resulting tendency toward hyperkalemia. Note that in the two renal tubular acidoses in which the distal tubule is the culprit, the quantity of hydrogen ion secreted is low; therefore, the patient has persistent acidosis, and urine pH will never be below 5.5 and is usually higher.

6

Elevated BUN/Creatinine Ratio

The BUN may rise disproportionately to creatinine by three mechanisms. The first mechanism has to do with the differences in the way the kidney handles filtered urea and filtered creatinine. Filtered creatinine passes through the renal tubules without being reabsorbed or secreted. Urea, on the other hand, because it is a nonpolar molecule and thus has the ability to cross plasma membranes in a passive manner, will move down a concentration gradient. Therefore, urea in renal tubules will be passively reabsorbed, and the extent of reabsorption will depend on its concentration in the tubule and the time it remains there. The higher the concentration and the longer it remains in the tubule the greater will be its reabsorption. The most frequent cause of a high BUN/creatinine ratio is volume depletion. In this condition, salt and water are avidly reabsorbed in the proximal tubule, thereby raising the concentration of urea in the tubule. Moreover, the urine flow through the tubule is quite slow. Obstructive uropathy will also cause a high BUN/creatinine ratio because the flow of glomerular filtrate through the kidneys is slow; therefore, urea remains in the tubules longer, and more of it is reabsorbed.

A second mechanism by which a high BUN/creatinine ratio occurs is increased delivery of amino acids to the liver. The liver makes urea out of amino acids; therefore, when an unusually large quantity of amino acids is delivered to the liver, it makes an unusually large quantity of urea. The most common cause of delivery of large quantities of amino acids to the liver is upper gastrointestinal hemorrhage: as the proteins in the blood are digested in the gut, a large load of amino acids is delivered to the liver. A second cause is catabolic states, in which an increased breakdown of muscle proteins results in the delivery of large quantities of amino acids to the liver.

The third mechanism by which an elevated BUN/creatinine ratio may occur is renal failure in a patient with very little muscle mass. Creatinine is generated by the breakdown of creatine from muscle. Patients with an inordinately small muscle mass will tend to have lower creatinine levels than they otherwise would have. Therefore, if they develop renal failure, the BUN will rise to an abnormal level but the creatinine may not. Thus, a BUN of 40 mg/dL and a creatinine of 1 mg/dL in an adult patient who weighs only 80 pounds and has very little muscle mass should lead the physician to consider that the BUN level, not the creatinine level, may more accurately reflect the patient's renal function. Measuring the creatinine clearance will resolve the issue.

7

Hypoglycemia

Hypoglycemia may occur by two general mechanisms: impaired glucose production and excessive insulin. Impaired glucose production occurs by three mechanisms: a deficiency of a hormone such as ACTH, cortisol, or growth hormone which boosts glucose levels; depletion of glycogen stores in severe malnutrition and in severe liver disease; and an inability to convert glycogen to glucose as occurs in ethanol and methanol intoxication and in genetic disorders of enzymes in the glycolytic pathway. The last mechanism generally causes glycogen storage diseases, so hypoglycemia by this mechanism is not usually a consideration in adults.

There are several mechanisms by which hypoglycemia may occur as a result of insulin excess. The two most common causes are an insulinoma and exogenous insulin administration. Less common causes include cytokine-mediated insulin production in sepsis, insulin "leak" from β-cell cytolysis by pentamidine, insulin production by sulfonylureas, production of insulin-like growth factor (IGF-2) by tumors, production of antibodies to insulin receptors in certain autoimmune diseases, and "reactive" hyperinsulinemia in dumping syndrome. In dumping syndrome, the delivery of a large bolus of glucose into the small bowel causes initial hyperglycemia followed by an overproduction of insulin with subsequent hypoglycemia.

The approach to the patient with hypoglycemia is first to document that glucose is low, by means of a 72-hour fast

TABLE 7.1
Mechanisms and Causes of Hypoglycemia

Underproduction of Glucose	Excessive Insulin

Hormone deficiency
  ACTH
  Cortisol
  Growth hormone
	Insulinoma

	Exogenous insulin administration
	Insulin receptor antibodies
Severe malnutrition	Sulfonylurea ingestion
Severe liver disease	Pentamidine administration

Alcohol intoxication
  Ethanol
  Methanol
	Sepsis

	IGF-2 production
Enzyme defect	Dumping syndrome

if necessary, and then to determine the insulin and C-peptide levels during hypoglycemia. All three determinations must be made on the same specimen of blood because an appropriate or inappropriate insulin level depends upon the glucose level. Low levels of insulin during hypoglycemia nearly always indicate that the mechanism of hypoglycemia is underproduction of glucose (see the exception below), and elevated insulin levels indicate excessive insulin. In the absence of excessive insulin, less than 10 grams per hour of glucose are required to maintain a normal blood glucose. Therefore, one hint that the mechanism of hypoglycemia is excessive insulin is the requirement of more than 10 grams of glucose per hour to maintain euglycemia in a hypoglycemic patient.

Once one has established that hypoglycemia is due to underproduction of glucose, making a specific diagnosis of liver disease, severe malnutrition, adrenal insufficiency, or pituitary failure should not be difficult, but ethanol and especially methanol intoxication may be less obvious. Likewise, insulin overproduction in sepsis, dumping syndrome, or pentamidine administration should be fairly obvious. The more challenging differential is to distinguish among insulinoma, exogenous insulin administration, sulfonylurea ingestion, IGF-2 production, and insulin receptor antibody production. If insulin levels during hypoglycemia are high and C-peptide is low, the diagnosis is exogenous insulin administration. If both insulin and C-peptide are high, then either the patient has an insulinoma, the patient has insulin receptor antibodies, or the patient has taken a sulfonyl-urea. If insulin and C-peptide are low, then IGF-2 production should be suspected.

Insulin receptor antibodies and IGF-2 production are quite rare, so the usual distinction is among insulinoma, exogenous insulin administration, and sulfonylurea ingestion. When patients are known to be taking insulin or a sulfonylurea, the diagnosis is usually easy. However, emotionally ill patients sometimes surreptitiously take insulin or a sulfonylurea, so a common challenge is distinguishing between self-administration of one of these agents and the presence of an insulinoma. Elevated insulin levels with low C-peptide levels establish the diagnosis of exogenously administered insulin. When both insulin and C-peptide levels are high, one should measure the blood sulfonylurea level to distinguish sulfonylurea administration from an insulinoma.

CLINICAL VIGNETTE

An 18-year-old woman with an emotional disorder that had manifested previously as manipulative behavior presented to the emergency room with a blood glucose of 20 mg/dL. Her mother, with whom she lived, was an insulin-requiring diabetic who had at times been taking a sulfonylurea. Even though the diagnosis of surreptitious self-administration of either insulin or sulfonylurea seemed obvious, the house-staff obtained simultaneous blood glucose, insulin, C-peptide, and sulfonylurea levels. At a time when the patient's serum glucose was 20 mg/dL, both her insulin and C-peptide levels were elevated, and the sulfonylurea level was 0. Subsequent evaluation revealed an insulinoma in the tail of the pancreas.

In this case, rather than relying on probability (the odds that the patient had surreptitiously taken either insulin or a sulfonylurea must have been at least 100 to 1), the house-staff reasoned thoroughly and pathophysiologically and disproved the "obvious" diagnosis and made the diagnosis of a very rare insulin-secreting tumor.

8

Osmolality

Osmolality is the "water-sucking power" of a molecule. It depends on the total number of particles in solution. One milliosmole (mOsm) is the water-sucking power of 1 millimole or 1 milliequivalent (mEq) of a substance. Most house officers know the formula for calculating serum osmolality: 2 times the serum concentration of sodium plus the serum glucose divided by 18 plus the BUN divided by 2.8. Not all house officers, however, understand or can derive that formula.

Once we understand the definition of osmolality, we can derive and analyze the formula. Sodium is a monovalent cation; it is the dominant cation in serum. All others are ignorable because they are present in such low concentrations relative to sodium. The serum sodium is expressed as mEq/L, so the osmolal force exerted by sodium is numerically the same as its concentration in mEq/L. That is, 1 mOsm/L is the same as 1 mEq/L. We multiply the serum sodium concentration by two to account for anions in the serum. The serum glucose is expressed as mg/dL. To obtain the osmolal force of glucose, we must divide the serum concentration by the milligram molecular weight, 180 mg/L. Because the numerator is expressed as mg/dL, we divide the denominator by 10 to make it similar, resulting in division of the serum value of glucose by 18. Similarly, BUN is expressed as mg/dL, and the molecular weight of urea is 28. Thus, 1 mOsm of urea would be 28 mg/L. Because the numerator is expressed as mg/dL, we divide the denominator by 10, resulting in division of the value of BUN by 2.8.

Note that, although albumin is quantitatively the most plentiful molecule in serum, we ignore it when calculating osmolality. It becomes obvious why we can ignore it if we include it in the formula. The serum concentration of albumin is about 4000 mg/dL or 40,000 mg/L. The molecular weight of albumin is about 60,000. Therefore, we have 40,000 mg/L in the numerator divided by the molecular weight of albumin, 60,000 mg/L, in the denominator. The result is less than 1 mOsm/L.

Thus, osmolality is the force exerted by molecules and it depends on the number of molecules in the serum. Even though large, plentiful molecules such as albumin dominate the concentration of substances in blood, they exert trivial osmolal force because they are so large that in terms of molality they are ignorable.

9

Hypercalcemia

Of the nine mechanisms by which hypercalcemia may occur, six are related to specific molecules. Parathormone (PTH) promotes hypercalcemia both by mobilizing the ion from bone and by enhancing its reabsorption in the kidney. Parathormone-related peptide (PTH-rP), secreted by epidermal tumors, promotes hypercalcemia in a manner similar to PTH. Osteoclast-activating factor, elaborated chiefly by myeloma cells, causes hypercalcemia by releasing the ion from bone. Thyroxine and vitamin A exert a direct effect on bone and sometimes cause mild hypercalcemia in hyperthyroidism and in massive vitamin A ingestion, respectively.

Vitamin D promotes hypercalcemia by enhancing its absorption from the gut. Hypervitaminosis D may occur as a result of ingestion of huge quantities of this vitamin. More commonly, however, vitamin D is produced in excess by activated macrophages in granulomatous diseases. The quantity of vitamin D produced depends on the number of activated macrophages and, therefore, on the number of granulomas. Of the granulomatous diseases, sarcoidosis is most commonly associated with hypervitaminosis D simply because among these diseases it is the one associated with the greatest number of granulomas. The mild hypercalcemia seen in adrenal insufficiency is due to the absence of normal suppression of the action of vitamin D by cortisol and therefore to enhanced absorption of calcium from the gut.

In milk-alkali syndrome the patient ingests large quantities of both calcium and alkali. The alkali markedly enhances absorption of calcium from the gut and reabsorption in the renal tubule. An alkaline environment enhances calcium absorption by driving more of the ion and its anion to the non-ionic state, allowing it to be passively absorbed like other nonpolar molecules such as urea. Thiazide diuretics block the secretion of calcium by the renal tubule. Finally, the immobilization of people who have bone diseases such as Paget's disease and occasionally the complete immobilization of other patients as well may result in disturbed calcium homeostasis, which may lead to hypercalcemia.

Of the routinely obtained laboratory studies, the serum phosphate level is probably the most helpful in differential diagnosis. It is low when the cause of hypercalcemia is PTH or PTH-rP; it is normal otherwise. The most important specific laboratory study is intact PTH at a time when serum calcium is elevated. The PTH is elevated when it is the cause of hypercalcemia; it is low in all other hypercalcemic states.

10

Hypocalcemia

The mechanisms by which hypocalcemia occurs are hypoparathyroidism, calcium binding to lipids in processes that result in saponification, calcium binding to phosphate in conditions causing very high serum phosphate levels, an elevated calcium–phosphorous product, and an unknown mechanism in toxic shock syndrome. Nearly every medical student and house officer knows that hypocalcemia occurs in pancreatitis because of fat necrosis and saponification of lipids. It is also important to know that hypocalcemia occurs with fat necrosis in other situations—for example, in necrotizing mixed aerobic–anaerobic soft tissue infections.

With toxic shock syndrome, the mechanism of hypocalcemia is still unknown. But the knowledge that it does occur is helpful diagnostically; for a patient who presents with a febrile illness characterized by rash and hypotension, the finding of hypocalcemia should strongly suggest toxic shock syndrome. Likewise, therapeutically, a patient with toxic shock syndrome is very likely to have hypocalcemia and require calcium replacement.

CLINICAL VIGNETTE

A 50-year-old diabetic man presented with progressive pain and erythema of the right leg that had persisted for 12 hours. The physical examination revealed only findings consistent with superficial cellulitis of the leg, which seemed to have begun at the site of a shallow ischemic ulcer. There was no evidence of abscess or of infection deeper than the skin.

Most of the screening laboratory data were consistent with what would be expected with cellulitis, but the house-staff noted a serum calcium level of 6 mg/dL (albumin and phosphate levels were normal). Quickly excluding most mechanisms of hypocalcemia, they realized that hypocalcemia in this clinical setting was most likely caused by fat necrosis. They obtained a radiograph of the leg, which revealed gas in the muscle. The patient was taken promptly to the operating room for exploration and débridement of necrotizing fasciitis and myositis.

With this patient there were no physical signs to suggest a deep necrotizing infection. The house-staff's understanding of the significance of hypocalcemia in this clinical setting led them to make the diagnosis quickly. Thus, they may well have not only saved the patient's leg, but even his life.

11

Hyperkalemia

Hyperkalemia may occur by five mechanisms. As potassium is the chief cation inside cells, one important cause of hyperkalemia is massive cellular destruction, such as occurs in tumor lysis syndrome or massive crush injuries. In acidosis, a second cause of hyperkalemia, potassium leaves the intracellular compartment in exchange for hydrogen ion; the resulting hyperkalemia is directly proportional to the degree of acidosis. Because potassium is filtered, reabsorbed, and then secreted by the renal tubule, renal failure resulting in inability to excrete sufficient quantities of potassium is a third important cause of hyperkalemia. Distal and Type IV RTAs result in the selective inability of the kidney to secrete potassium, and thus they are a fourth cause of hyperkalemia; trimethoprim and pentamidine can cause hyperkalemia by inducing Type IV RTA. Finally, in primary or secondary hypoaldosteronism, potassium cannot be exchanged for sodium and secreted by the distal tubule, thus making it the fifth cause of hyperkalemia. Angiotensin-converting enzyme (ACE) inhibitors and nonsteroidal anti-inflammatory drugs (NSAIDs) cause hyperkalemia by impairing aldosterone secretion (primary hypoaldosteronism) and renal potassium secretion (secondary hypoaldosteronism), respectively.

12

Hyperphosphatemia

There are only four causes of an elevated serum phosphate level. The most common cause is renal failure, which is never a diagnostic dilemma. The second most common cause is acidosis, where both phosphate and potassium leave the intracellular compartment for the extracellular compartment. In acidosis, the total body phosphate stores are often low, in spite of the elevated serum determination, because phosphate is lost in the urine (for example, by osmotic diuresis in diabetes). The third cause is massive tissue destruction, which is most commonly seen in so-called tumor lysis syndrome in which lysis of a huge tumor load by treatment with chemotherapeutic agents results in the release of intracellular materials including phosphate. The fourth cause is hypoparathyroidism.

CLINICAL VIGNETTE

An elderly woman was brought to the hospital by her family simply because she "didn't seem quite right." The physical examination was totally unremarkable. Her laboratory evaluation was similarly normal except for a serum phosphate of 13 mg/dL, which was again 13 mg/dL when repeated on a different specimen of blood. That laboratory determination led to her admission. The house-staff was initially quite puzzled. However, because they understood the mechanisms by which phosphate could become elevated, they reasoned logically and came to the correct diagnosis.

There was no evidence that the patient was hypoparathyroid. Determination of arterial blood gases excluded acidosis. She did not have renal failure. They reasoned that the only mechanism left was massive tissue destruction. There was nothing to suggest tumor lysis syndrome, and she had not sustained an injury that might have resulted in massive tissue destruction. The house-staff reasoned that the only source of massive tissue necrosis that could be so clinically inapparent would be in the abdomen. They obtained a computed tomography (CT) scan of her abdomen, which revealed necrosis of the entire small and large bowel. Soon the patient developed the typical signs and laboratory manifestations of necrotic bowel: abdominal pain, distention, and tenderness in conjunction with sepsis and lactic acidosis. She died shortly thereafter.

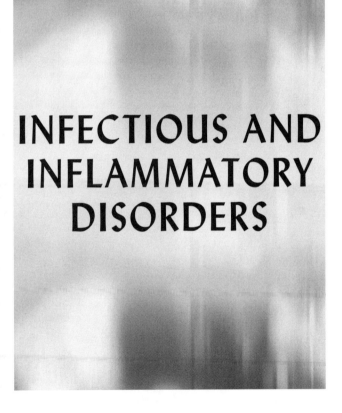

P A R T

II

INFECTIOUS AND INFLAMMATORY DISORDERS

13

Erythrocyte Sedimentation Rate

To describe the physiology of an elevated erythrocyte sedimentation rate (ESR), I will initially reason backward from the test itself. Then I will summarize the physiology going forward.

The ESR is determined by a very simple test. One simply draws blood into a capillary tube or some other tube marked from 0 to roughly 150 mm. Once the column of blood has been filled to the highest mark (the 0 mark), the other end of the tube is sealed, and the tube is allowed to stand vertically for an hour. After an hour the technologist simply reads the number of millimeters that the erythrocytes have fallen. The normal ESR is low, only 10 to 20 mm per hour. That is because, like other cells, erythrocyte surfaces are negatively charged and repel each other, thereby preventing agglutination.

An elevated ESR occurs when a protein or proteins, which are both positively and negatively charged, are present in high concentrations in the serum and coat the erythrocytes. As the erythrocyte surfaces become both positively and negatively charged, they attract each other and fall rapidly, resulting in an elevated ESR. One such protein responsible for agglutinating erythrocytes is a monoclonal immunoglobulin (Ig) or light chain in multiple myeloma. More commonly, so-called acute phase reactants are responsible. These include numerous proteins such as serum amyloid protein A, β_2-microglobulin, haptoglobin, complement proteins, ceruloplasmin, transferrin, and C-reactive protein. These proteins are produced by hepatocytes in response to elaboration of cytokines, most particularly interleukin-6 (IL-6), by macrophages. Macrophages produce IL-6 when any of a number of their cell surface receptors are engaged by infectious or inflammatory products. These cell surface molecules include the receptors for the Fc portion of IgG, for the third component of complement, for γ-interferon, for lipoteichoic acid of gram-positive bacteria, for lipopolysaccharide of gram-negative bacteria, for mannan of fungi, for "cord factors" of mycobacteria, and for double-stranded RNA of viruses.

Thus, infection with gram-positive or gram-negative bacteria, mycobacteria, fungi, or viruses produces products that engage the appropriate receptors on the surfaces of macrophages. In addition, sterile inflammation caused by cell-mediated immunity (γ-interferon receptor) or by immune complex disease (IgG Fc receptor and C3 receptor) produces molecules that similarly engage receptors on the surfaces of macrophages. Engagement of any of these receptors activates the macrophages' genes for a number of products, including IL-6. IL-6 binds to the surfaces of hepatocytes and causes the hepatocytes to turn off the gene for albumin and to activate genes for acute phase reactants. These acute phase reactants bind to the surfaces of erythrocytes and, as they are both positively and negatively charged, cause the erythrocytes to agglutinate, resulting in an elevated ESR.

Thus, an elevated ESR means that the patient is experiencing an active infectious or noninfectious inflammatory process or that the patient has multiple myeloma.

14

Acute Undifferentiated Fever

Acute undifferentiated fever, or acute fever of unknown origin (FUO), is one of the most intellectually challenging conditions a physician can face. A patient, often one who was quite healthy until hours or a few days earlier, presents with an illness of fairly short duration characterized by fever but without any symptoms or signs pointing either to the location of the problem or to the causative agent. Such a disorder usually has three major mechanisms: infection with microorganisms, immune complex deposition, and/or thermoregulatory disorders. By far the most important of these is infection with microorganisms.

It is mandatory that the physician understand acute undifferentiated fever and have a plan of approach in mind before encountering such patients because acute undifferentiated fever can present as or can rapidly become acute overwhelming sepsis. Thus, the physician must know every microorganism that can cause such a disorder so that empiric therapy, which must be initiated immediately with an ill patient, will include a drug effective against the offending pathogen.

I do not know any way to use reasoning to generate a list of organisms that can cause acute undifferentiated fever. Table 14.1 is a list of such organisms by their taxonomic classification. The first five pathogens are bacteria

TABLE 14.1
Microbial Causes of Acute Undifferentiated Fever

Bacteria	Viruses	Protozoa
Common	**Infectious Mononucleosis**	*Plasmodium*
Staphylococcus aureus	**Group**	species
Streptococcus	Epstein-Barr virus	*Babesia*
pneumoniae	Cytomegalovirus	species
Streptococcus pyogenes	Hepatitis A virus	*Toxoplasma*
Neisseria meningitidis	Hepatitis B virus	*gondii*
Haemophilus influenzae	Hepatitis C virus	
Uncommon	Human immunodeficiency	
Clostridium species	virus	
Yersinia pestis	**Rodent-borne/Arbovirus**	
Pseudomonas	**Group**	
pseudomallei	Dengue	
Vibrio vulnificus	Colorado tick fever	
Capnocytophaga	Hantaan virus	
canimorsus	Marburg virus	
Salmonella species	Ebola virus	
Yersinia species	Hemorrhagic fever viruses	
Brucella species	Venezuelan equine	
Campylobacter species	encephalomyelitis virus	
Francisella tularensis	**Childhood Exanthem**	
Chlamydia psittaci	**Viruses**	
Legionella species	Measles virus	
Rickettsiae	Varicella virus	
Coxiella burnetii	Parvovirus B19	
Rickettsia prowazekii		
Rickettsia rickettsii		
Ehrlichia species		
Spirochetes		
Leptospira species		
Borrelia recurrentis		

that commonly cause acute undifferentiated fever and often cause acute overwhelming sepsis. In a patient with acute sepsis, empiric therapy should include coverage against all of these microorganisms. The next five are less common causes, but these organisms can also overwhelm a healthy patient within hours. If there is epidemiologic evidence to suggest infection with any of them, they also should be covered by initial empiric therapy.

The next five organisms in Table 14.1 include *Salmonella* and others that cause so-called enteric fever. These organisms would not overwhelm a patient within hours, but they can make a patient dreadfully ill within days. In a patient who presents with an illness that has lasted several days and is septic, these organisms should be considered and perhaps treated empirically as well.

The next three organisms listed in Table 14.1 are inhaled, and are typically associated with atypical pneumonia syndrome. However, after they have landed in the alveoli, these organisms home into the reticuloendothelial system where they replicate during the first several days of illness and may cause acute FUO before causing a pulmonary infiltrate.

The Rickettsiae and *Ehrlichia* species can also overwhelm a healthy patient, although they generally require several days to a week to do so. They should also be considered and treated empirically in a patient who is septic after an illness of several days' duration. The two spirochetes listed are uncommon causes of acute undifferentiated fever.

Most viral illnesses do not cause undifferentiated fever; rather, they cause respiratory symptoms or sometimes gastrointestinal symptoms. There are three exceptions. Acute undifferentiated fever is the usual presenting syndrome in infectious mononucleosis syndrome, illnesses caused by the rodent-borne/arbovirus group of viruses, and occasionally the childhood exanthem diseases. These latter viruses may cause undifferentiated fever for 12 to 24 hours before the onset of a typical rash.

Of the protozoa, *Toxoplasma gondii* can cause a mononucleosis-like illness, presenting as acute undifferentiated fever syndrome. Malaria and babesia are also protozoa that typically cause acute undifferentiated fever.

CLINICAL VIGNETTE

A 20-year-old woman presented with a 36-hour history of progressively severe malaise, fever, weakness, and rash. The physical examination revealed a moderately ill woman whose blood pressure was 105/50, temperature was 101°F (38.3°C), and heart rate 105. She had a diffuse erythematous rash. The BUN, creatinine, aspartate aminotransferase (AST), bilirubin, and alkaline phosphatase levels were all moderately elevated, each about twice the upper limits of normal. Her serum calcium level was 6 mg/dL (albumin and phosphate levels were normal).

Although the differential diagnosis was quite broad and the house-staff were prepared to treat the patient broadly for sepsis, the combination of rash, hypotension, multi-organ disease, and especially hypocalcemia led them to consider toxic shock syndrome (TSS). They took a careful menstrual history and learned that the patient had just that morning completed an especially heavy menstrual period requiring her to use superabsorbent tampons.

The patient recovered uneventfully after treatment with an anti-staphylococcal penicillin and clindamycin, the latter to impair the production of TSS toxin. The blood cultures remained sterile; the vaginal culture eventually grew *Staphylococcus aureus*.

The brevity and severity of the patient's illness suggested sepsis with a bacterium that is capable of quickly overwhelming even a healthy patient (see the first 10 organisms listed in Table 14.1). The rash and hypocalcemia led the house-staff to consider TSS specifically, and to probe further into the history to obtain evidence in support of that diagnosis.

15

Chronic Fever of Undetermined Origin

For a process to cause fever without important focal symptoms or signs, it must be in the intravascular system, in the abdomen or retroperitoneum, or in the reticuloendothelial system, areas that can house a pathologic condition without causing local symptoms and are not easily accessible by physical examination. The differential diagnosis of fever of undetermined origin (FUO) has changed considerably in the past several decades, and now depends upon at what point in the evaluation one defines the FUO. As CT scanning has become the first major test used in approaching patients with FUO, conditions such as intra-abdominal abscess can now be immediately identified or eliminated as FUO causes.

The major differential diagnostic categories of FUO are infection, collagen vascular disease, and neoplasia. In the United States, infections that cause chronic fever include tuberculosis, histoplasmosis, infectious endocarditis, and intra-abdominal bacterial infection. Elsewhere in the world, kala-azar, Q fever, and brucellosis are additional causes. Very few other infectious diseases cause chronic fever. Of the immunologic inflammatory diseases, juvenile rheumatoid arthritis in a 25 year old patient, polyarteritis nodosa in a 50-year-old patient, and giant cell arteritis in a 75-year-old patient most commonly present as FUO. Occasionally systemic lupus erythematosus and drug fever present as FUO.

Less common causes may be inflammatory bowel disease, sarcoidosis, and immunologic liver disease. Other primary immunologic diseases such as rheumatoid arthritis and Wegener's granulomatosis rarely cause FUO because they present with focal symptoms or signs.

Three neoplasms—lymphoma/Hodgkin's disease, renal cell carcinoma, and hepatoma—cause FUO by elaborating interleukin-1. Other tumors only rarely present as FUO; when they cause fever, it is generally because they have obstructed an important passage and caused infection behind that obstruction. For example, lung cancer can obstruct a bronchus, or bladder cancer a ureter. Other causes of FUO are extraordinarily uncommon; one such extraordinary cause is featured in the clinical vignette.

CLINICAL VIGNETTE

A 40-year-old Chilean man presented to the infectious diseases clinic after having had repeated episodes of fever. He was asymptomatic at the time, but over the past 15 to 20 years he had had 10 to 15 febrile episodes, each exactly like the others. The illnesses would begin abruptly with chills, fever, and malaise. These symptoms would worsen over 2 to 3 days and subside within 7 to 10 days, either spontaneously or after treatment with antibiotics. He had never had any symptoms other than the chills, fever, and malaise; between episodes of illness he was entirely asymptomatic and was able to continue the world travels related to his job as an importer of exotic goods in Santiago.

The physical examination revealed nothing remarkable at the time of presentation. By his history and the medical records he brought from his Santiago physicians, the examination during each of the previous episodes likewise had been unremarkable. The blood cultures, screening laboratory data, bone marrow examinations, CT scans of the chest and abdomen, and numerous serologic tests for exotic infectious diseases and for non-infectious immunologic diseases had revealed nothing remarkable.

The clinic physician reasoned that both neoplastic disease and immunologic disease seemed excluded by the duration over which the patient's episodes had occurred, by the lack of evidence of progressive or chronic disease, and by his being completely normal between episodes. Repeated or relapsing infectious diseases seemed improbable. The lack of any signs of the usual causes of FUO in the three major categories led the physician to consider unusual disorders that might occur repeatedly but infrequently, taking no chronic toll on the patient.

With familial Mediterranean fever specifically in mind, the physician asked the patient about his ethnic background. The patient revealed that, although he was Chilean, his genetic roots were in Syria. In fact, the patient's cousin had classic familial Mediterranean fever. The patient had not considered that he himself might have that disorder simply because he had never had peritonitis during his episodes. The physician could assure the patient that he had familial Mediterranean fever, and that further evaluation for other causes of fever was not indicated. The relative infrequency of his episodes made prophylactic treatment with an agent such as colchicine unnecessary, and he was advised to have the individual episodes treated symptomatically.

16

Infections in Immunocompromised Patients

There are three limbs of cellular host defense: neutrophils, B lymphocytes, and T lymphocytes/macrophages. When an organism invades our tissues, we marshall all three cellular host defenses against the invader: neutrophils rush to the site; B lymphocytes are triggered by microbial antigens to replicate, differentiate, and begin to elaborate specific IgG antibody against the pathogen; and T lymphocytes are similarly triggered to differentiate, expand, and become activated to elaborate lymphokines, most notably γ-interferon, which activate macrophages. In essentially every case, however, two out of three of these responses are unnecessary—only one determines the outcome of the encounter between the host and the pathogen.

The microorganisms that each of these cellular host defense limbs defend against have similar characteristics. Neutrophils defend us against organisms that are easy to eat and easy to kill; IgG antibody defends us against organisms that are hard to eat but easy to kill; and the T lymphocyte/macrophage system, or the cell-mediated immune system, defends us against organisms that are easy to eat but hard to kill. As we will see, there is a nearly perfect correlation between what we find when we study microbe–cell interactions in vitro and what we find in vivo with patients who have defects in a particular cellular defense mechanism.

After circulating for a few hours in the bloodstream, neutrophils emigrate into tissues, especially the lamina propria of the gastrointestinal tract through which they wander on their way to die in the gut lumen. Every day small numbers of our own gastrointestinal flora get through the mucosa and into the lamina propria. A few of these organisms even get into our bloodstream. An important role of neutrophils is to patrol these submucosal areas and to ingest and destroy these invading microorganisms. Having neutrophils, therefore, allows us to coexist with our own normal flora, chiefly enteric gram-negative bacilli, enterococci, and staphylococci.

When patients are hospitalized and placed on antimicrobial agents, their gut flora change to more resistant gram-negative bacilli, yeasts, and even molds such as *Aspergillus*. All of these microorganisms share a common interaction with neutrophils. If one incubates them in a Petri dish on which normal neutrophils have been plated, the microbes will be readily engulfed and destroyed. They are not encapsulated and thus present no barrier to phagocytosis; nor are they well equipped to survive within a phagocytic cell. Neutrophils, then, are our necessary and sufficient defenders against this group of pathogens. When neutrophils are either deficient in number or defective in function, organisms that cross the mucosa and make their way into the lamina propria encounter no neutrophils to destroy them and are able to proliferate and to cause local disease. They may cause a contiguous infection or a distant infection by bacteremia. Table 16.1 identifies the pathogens that infect patients with neutrophil dysfunction.

The major function of the humoral immune system is to produce IgG antibody, whose main defensive action against infection is to coat, or opsonize, microorganisms that are not readily ingested. Most of these microorganisms are not ingestible because they express a capsule on their surfaces for which phagocytic cells have no surface receptors. The prototypes of such organisms are *Streptococcus pneumoniae*

TABLE 16.1
Microorganisms Causing Infection in Patients
with Neutrophil Disorders

Staphylococcus aureus
Enterococci
Streptococci
Enteric gram-negative bacilli
Pseudomonas aeruginosa
Candida
Aspergillus

TABLE 16.2
Microorganisms Infecting Patients with Defects in Humoral Immunity

Streptococcus pneumoniae
Haemophilus influenzae
Encapsulated strains of gram-negative bacilli

---

and *Haemophilus influenzae*. However, a small percentage of enteric gram-negative bacilli and even a few strains of *Staphylococcus aureus* express capsules as well. When one incubates encapsulated pneumococci in a Petri dish coated with a monolayer of either neutrophils or macrophages, the phagocytic cells fail to ingest the bacteria. However, when in a companion Petri dish one offers the phagocytes IgG-coated pneumococci, the bacteria are readily engulfed; because they are ill-equipped to survive within the cell, they are rapidly killed. Assuming there is no phagocytic defect, IgG is the necessary and sufficient host defense mechanism protecting us against infection with organisms that are hard to ingest but easy to kill. Table 16.2 lists the micro-organisms that infect patients with humoral immune defects; they are the organisms predicted by the in vitro findings to infect these patients.

Table 16.3 lists the microorganisms that cause infections in patients who have defects in the cell-mediated immune system. Despite their taxonomic diversity, these pathogens do share a common feature. When offered to a monolayer of macrophages in a Petri dish, these micro-

TABLE 16.3
Microorganisms Causing Infection in Patients
with Defective Cell-mediated Immunity

Bacteria	Viruses
Mycobacteria	Herpes simplex virus
Legionella	Varicella zoster virus
Listeria monocytogenes	Cytomegalovirus
Nocardia asteroides	Epstein-Barr virus
Rhodococcus equi	Polyoma viruses
Bartonella henselae	Adenoviruses

Fungi	Parasites
Cryptococcus neoformans	Pneumocystis carinii
Histoplasma capsulatum	Toxoplasma gondii
Coccidioides immitis	Strongyloides stercoralis
Blastomyces dermatitidis	Cryptosporidium parvum
Candida (mucosal)	Isospora belli
Aspergillus	

organisms are readily ingested; however, once they are inside the macrophage, they cannot be killed and will often replicate within the cell and completely destroy the monolayer. Yet these organisms can be eaten and readily killed—or are at least considerably inhibited within the cell—by macrophages that have been previously treated with γ-interferon, thereby having their killing capabilities markedly enhanced. As in the Petri dish, patients who are unable to activate their macrophages are susceptible to infection with these intracellular pathogens.

Understanding these principles of the cellular host defense system enables physicians to consider the appropriate infectious agents in a patient who has a specific cellular host defense defect. Appropriate empiric therapy can be selected if a specific microbial diagnosis is not apparent at the outset, and rational decisions can be made regarding whether and when to perform an invasive diagnostic procedure. For example, in patients with neutrophil defects or with humoral immune defects, an infection is generally caused by a limited number of bacteria. We can provide effective empiric therapy with two or three antimicrobial agents, and we have a reasonable prospect of making a specific diagnosis from a culture within 24 hours. In contrast, patients with cell-mediated immune defects could be infected with a host of microorganisms, making empiric therapy impractical. Moreover, many of these microorganisms never grow in culture or grow very slowly. Thus, to more readily target their therapy, these patients often require invasive procedures to obtain biopsy material for making a specific diagnosis.

CLINICAL VIGNETTE

A 65-year-old woman who had been receiving high-dose prednisone for 2 months to treat IgA nephropathy presented to the hospital with chills, fever, malaise, and mild headache that had become progressively more severe over the past 24 hours. Except for a fever of 102°F (39°C), her physical examination was unremarkable. Her white blood cell count (WBC) was 14,000/μL. Because she was receiving prednisone, the patient was at risk for infection with the microorganisms listed in Table 16.3. The house-staff reasoned that viral, parasitic, fungal, and mycobacterial disease were very unlikely because of the brevity of the patient's illness. They therefore focused on the remaining opportunistic bacteria; the only one that typically causes acute undifferentiated fever is *Listeria*.

Because the patient had a headache, albeit mild, and because *Listeria* bacteremia often results in meningoencephalitis, they performed a lumbar puncture. The patient's cerebrospinal fluid (CSF) revealed 50 neutrophils/μL and a slightly elevated protein level; the gram stain was non-revealing. The house-staff included ampicillin in their initial empiric antibiotic regimen, and the patient's symptoms promptly resolved. Subsequently, the patient's blood and CSF both grew *Listeria monocytogenes*.

The house-staff in this case focused on the microorganisms shown in Table 16.3 because they understood the nature of this patient's underlying immunologic defect, impairment of cell-mediated immunity by prednisone, and had familiarity with the spectrum of microbial pathogens that tend to infect such patients. They focused on a specific subset of bacterial pathogens because they knew that the brevity of the patient's illness made fungal, viral, parasitic, and mycobacterial infections unlikely. They performed a lumbar puncture because they were aware of *Listeria*'s propensity for homing to the central nervous system, and they included empiric therapy for *Listeria* from the outset.

17

Cerebrospinal Fluid Pleocytosis

When we discover leukocytes in the CSF, we often make the diagnosis of meningitis. It is important, however, to understand that cells may gain access to the CSF not only by meningeal inflammation but also by processes in or adjacent to the brain and spinal cord. CSF pleocytosis may occur by three other mechanisms: encephalitis, vasculitis, and parameningeal foci of bacterial infection. Thus, the physician must be very careful and very circumspect in elucidating the cause of CSF pleocytosis.

High fever, a rigid neck, and confusion are signs of meningeal inflammation. Confusion and focal neurologic signs out of proportion to nuchal rigidity should lead the physician to consider not only encephalitis or cerebral vasculitis as the cause of CSF pleocytosis, but also focal bacterial processes such as a brain abscess, subdural empyema, or epidural abscess. In these days of nearly universal use of imaging studies, it is highly unlikely that we will be confused by these parameningeal infectious foci in the cranium. However, a spinal epidural abscess may be more easily missed, so the physician needs to be particularly attentive to even subtle neurologic signs that may suggest this diagnosis in a patient with CSF pleocytosis.

18

Neutrophilic Cerebrospinal Fluid Pleocytosis

The finding of neutrophilic CSF pleocytosis leads the physician appropriately to entertain a diagnosis of bacterial meningitis and in most situations to treat for that disorder empirically. That is certainly the appropriate approach. However, it is important to understand that there are several other mechanisms and many additional causes of neutrophilic CSF pleocytosis. The four mechanisms are local infections, certain systemic infections, noninfectious local inflammatory disorders, and noninfectious systemic inflammatory diseases (Table 18.1).

In addition to bacterial meningitis, several other infections can cause a predominantly neutrophilic CSF pleocytosis. These include viral meningitis during the first 24 hours of illness; tuberculous meningitis, especially during therapy when products from lysing tubercle bacilli attract neutrophils into the CSF; blastomycotic meningitis; *Naegleria* meningoencephalitis; and, surprisingly, cytomegalovirus (CMV) myelitis in AIDS patients. A brain abscess, subdural empyema, or epidural abscess usually causes a pleocytosis that is an approximately equal mixture of neutrophils and mononuclear cells; however, if the abscess abuts the ventricle or the meninges (as it does perhaps 5% to 10% of the

TABLE 18.1
Mechanisms and Causes of Neutrophilic CSF Pleocytosis

Local Infections	*Sterile Local Inflammation*
Bacterial meningitis	Blood
Early viral meningitis	Air
Tuberculous meningitis on treatment	Myelography dye
	Locally injected drugs
Blastomycotic meningitis	Cyst rupture into CSF
Naegleria meningoencephalitis	*Sterile Systemic Inflammation*
CMV myelitis in AIDS	Systemic lupus erythematosus
Parameningeal infection	Behçet's disease
Systemic Infections	Primary CNS vasculitis
Rocky Mountain spotted fever	Drugs such as NSAIDs
Epidemic typhus	
Staphylococcal bacteremia	

time), the CSF formula may look exactly like that of bacterial meningitis. Because patients with fever and signs suggesting a central nervous system infection nearly always undergo brain imaging studies, it would be most unusual for these abscesses to be missed and the patient thought to have meningitis only.

In addition to local infections, systemic infection with *Rickettsiae*, most particularly with the causative agent of Rocky Mountain spotted fever (RMSF), and bacteremia, most especially staphylococcal bacteremia, result in deposition of microorganisms either in capillary endothelial cells (RSMF) or in capillaries throughout the brain (staphylococcal bacteremia). Patients may therefore have an "encephalitis" or cerebral vasculitis due to these systemic infections. Sometimes the central nervous system involvement may cause a patient to present predominantly as someone with a primary brain or meningeal infection. If the physician is not attuned to the possibility of RMSF or staphylococcal bacteremia presenting with predominantly neurologic symptoms, then the neutrophilic CSF pleocytosis may be misinterpreted and the patient treated only for the usual causes of bacterial meningitis, which may not include therapy for either of these disorders.

Neutrophilic CSF pleocytosis may occur in response to local irritants. Blood, air, myelography dye, other drugs injected into the subarachnoid space, and the contents of brain cysts or craniopharyngiomas when they rupture into the subarachnoid space are very irritating to the meninges. The substances elicit an intense inflammatory response characterized by large numbers of neutrophils, moderate elevations in protein, and sometimes hypoglycorrhachia as well, often exactly mimicking the CSF findings in bacterial meningitis.

Sterile inflammation of the brain as a manifestation of several systemic disorders is a final mechanism by which neutrophilic CSF pleocytosis may occur. Diseases such as systemic lupus erythematosus, Behçet's disease, primary central nervous system vasculitis, and meningitis caused by drugs such as NSAIDs are examples of diseases causing neutrophilic pleocytosis by this mechanism.

CLINICAL VIGNETTE

The Infectious Diseases service was asked to see a 50-year-old man because of meningitis. He had been admitted obtunded with fever and stiff neck 3 days earlier. His CSF had revealed 3000 neutrophils/μL, a glucose level of 15 mg/dL, and protein level of 700 mg/dL. Neither the gram stain or culture of CSF nor the blood cultures had revealed an organism, and the patient was only slightly improved after 3 days of treatment with appropriate antibiotics.

The Infectious Diseases fellow reviewed the chart carefully and noted that, in addition to the leukocyte, glucose, and protein abnormalities of the CSF, the laboratory had reported a red blood cell (RBC) count of 30,000/μL and had noted that the CSF was strikingly xanthochromic. When asked about these findings, the primary physician said he had assumed that the erythrocytes were due to a traumatic lumbar puncture. The fellow asked the patient's family about the onset and progress of his illness. The family said that the patient had been perfectly normal until the morning of presentation to the hospital when he had experienced the abrupt onset of headache and became progressively obtunded over 2 hours. The patient's history, the bloody and xanthochromic CSF, the absence of an organism in the CSF, and the failure of the patient to respond to antibacterial therapy strongly suggested that the patient had sustained a subarachnoid hemorrhage. Arteriography revealed a ruptured berry aneurysm.

On the surface it may seem absurd that subarachnoid hemorrhage could be confused with bacterial meningitis. However, on at least five occasions over the past several years I have encountered exactly the situation described above. Traumatic lumbar punctures are fairly common, leading us sometimes to dismiss even substantial numbers of erythrocytes in CSF as being caused by the lumbar puncture itself. Moreover, the presence of several thousand neutrophils, of hypoglycorrhachia, and of strikingly elevated protein appropriately alert the physician to the probability that the patient has bacterial meningitis, and it is certainly prudent to treat for bacterial meningitis in such a situation. However, it is important to realize that numerous other disorders, including those listed in Table 18.1, can cause neutrophilic CSF pleocytosis and to pay special attention to the temporal profile of a patient's illness, to the presence of erythrocytes in the CSF, and most especially, to the finding of xanthochromia in CSF (see Chapter 20). Doing so in this case led the Infectious Diseases fellow to the correct diagnosis.

19

Lymphocytic Cerebrospinal Fluid Pleocytosis

When we attempt to elucidate the cause of CSF pleocytosis that is dominantly lymphocytic, it is helpful to divide the causes into those that normally cause and those that normally do not cause hypoglycorrhachia. The mechanism by which CSF glucose becomes depressed is interference with the glucose transporter in the choroid plexus that is responsible for pumping glucose from the ependymal cells into the ventricular fluid. In certain inflammatory disorders, usually those primarily affecting the meninges as opposed to the brain substance itself, there is presumably a substance formed that "poisons" the glucose transporter.

There are five causes of lymphocytic CSF pleocytosis with hypoglycorrhachia (Table 19.1). They are tuberculous meningitis, fungal meningitis, sarcoidosis of the central nervous system, partially treated bacterial meningitis, and meningeal carcinomatosis. Note that the pathologic condition in each of these disorders is centered primarily or exclusively in the meninges themselves.

The causes of lymphocytic CSF pleocytosis with normal glucose are more numerous (see Table 19.1). They include viral meningitis and encephalitis, and three spirochetal infections that closely mimic viral infection of the CNS:

TABLE 19.1
Mechanisms and Causes of Lymphocytic CSF Pleocytosis

Low Glucose	Normal Glucose
Tuberculosis	Numerous viruses
Fungal meningitis	Meningitis
Cryptococcus neoformans	Encephalitis
Coccidioides immitis	Spirochetes
Sarcoidosis	Syphilis
Partially treated	Leptospirosis
bacterial meningitis	Lyme disease
Meningeal carcinomatosis	Vasculitis
	Systemic lupus erythematosus
	Behçet's disease
	Primary CNS vasculitis
	Parameningeal infections
	Brain abscess
	Subdural empyema
	Epidural abscess

syphilis, leptospirosis, and Lyme disease. Another cause is vasculitis, including all of the causes discussed in the preceding chapter. Vasculitis may result in predominantly neutrophils or predominantly mononuclear cells in the CSF. Finally, parameningeal bacterial infections—brain abscess, subdural empyema, and epidural abscess—typically cause CSF inflammation with a roughly equal number of lymphocytes and neutrophils. Thus, in any given patient, neutrophils may predominate or lymphocytes may predominate.

20

Evaluating Cerebrospinal Fluid That Contains Erythrocytes

When the physician learns that the CSF obtained from performing a lumbar puncture contains erythrocytes, every effort must be made to determine whether those erythrocytes were present in the CSF or were introduced by trauma from the lumbar puncture itself. Moreover, physicians must know how to properly interpret the results of the WBC count and the protein determinations on the specimen containing erythrocytes.

It seems to have become routine to send the first and last tubes of CSF for the cell count; a decrease in the RBC count between the first and last tubes is seen as evidence that erythrocytes are present as a consequence of a traumatic lumbar puncture, or similar RBC counts in the first and last tubes are seen as evidence that erythrocytes were present in the CSF. I find this procedure of very limited value, as it often diverts attention away from a more critical appraisal that would yield much more important information.

Because only 200 erythrocytes/μL are required to discolor CSF, even tiny quantities of blood in the CSF will be easily detected by visual examination of the fluid. When the final tube of collected CSF is crystal clear, then I believe only that tube need be sent for the cell count. If earlier tubes were discolored by blood, then it is obvious that the blood was introduced by a traumatic lumbar puncture. When all tubes are crystal clear, then we are not likely to attach much significance to any erythrocytes that may be present because they will be so few. Only when both the first and last tubes are discolored will sending both tubes for RBC count provide useful information.

Much more important, however, in trying to determine the source of erythrocytes in CSF is to determine whether the supernatant of centrifuged CSF is xanthochromic. When the last tube of collected CSF is discolored, the physician should immediately centrifuge it and examine the supernatant. It takes only a few hours for erythrocytes present in CSF to lyse, rendering the fluid xanthochromic. Thus, if centrifuged CSF is not xanthochromic, one can reasonably conclude that the source of erythrocytes in the fluid is either from a traumatic lumbar puncture or from a very recent bleed into the CSF. The clinical situation should enable the physician to distinguish between these possibilities.

It is important that the physician understand how to properly evaluate the WBC count and the protein determination of CSF that contains erythrocytes, especially if those erythrocytes were introduced via a traumatic lumbar puncture. When blood is introduced into CSF via a traumatic lumbar puncture, the number of leukocytes and the quantity of protein introduced along with erythrocytes will be exactly proportional to their relationship to erythrocytes in blood. If leukocytes or protein were present in excessive quantity in the CSF, then their numbers will be disproportionately elevated in comparison to the number of erythrocytes introduced via the traumatic lumbar puncture. To determine the number of leukocytes or the quantity of protein that can be accounted for by a traumatic lumbar puncture, one need simply set up a ratio equation such as that in Figure 20.1: the number of erythrocytes in CSF divided by the number of erythrocytes in peripheral blood is compared with the number of leukocytes in the CSF divided by the number of leukocytes in peripheral blood. One can establish a similar equation to determine the quantity of protein

FIGURE 20.1

$$\frac{\text{WBC (CSF)}}{\text{WBC (Blood)}} = \frac{\text{RBC (CSF)}}{\text{RBC (Blood)}}$$

$$\frac{\text{Protein (CSF)}}{\text{Protein (Blood)}} = \frac{\text{RBC (CSF)}}{\text{RBC (Blood)}}$$

Determining the significance of CSF WBC counts and protein determinations in CSF containing blood. Insert the laboratory values for WBC (Blood), Protein (Blood), RBC (CSF), and RBC (Blood) and solve for WBC (CSF) and Protein (CSF). Then compare the calculated values with the measured values for WBC (CSF) and Protein (CSF).

that can be accounted for by a traumatic lumbar puncture. As a general rule, 1 leukocyte/μL can be accounted for by 1000 erythrocytes/μL, and about 0.7 mg/dL of protein can be accounted for by 1000 erythrocytes/μL. However, because the number of erythrocytes and leukocytes in the peripheral blood of a given individual can be markedly different from the average upon which the above-stated rule of thumb is based, it is important that the physician critically evaluate the significance of leukocytes and protein in the CSF by solving the equations for each patient. For practice, the reader may wish to use the values for the CSF abnormalities of the patient discussed in the clinical vignette of Chapter 18 to determine whether the leukocytes and protein in his CSF could have been accounted for simply by a traumatic lumbar puncture. Assume that his peripheral RBC count was 5 million/μL, his peripheral WBC count was 5000/μL, and his serum protein was 7 grams/dL.

CARDIOVASCULAR AND PULMONARY DISORDERS

21

Dyspnea

There are only three mechanisms responsible for eliciting the sensation of dyspnea: acidosis, J receptor stimulation, and central triggering of the respiratory center in the medulla.

We have all experienced the sensation of dyspnea. All physiologic states that involve exertion generate quantities of lactic acid that cannot be immediately metabolized, resulting in lactic acidosis that may drop our pH to 7.0 or below. Once exertion stops, the lactate is rapidly metabolized and the sensation of dyspnea resolves. Pathologic states that result in acidosis likewise cause dyspnea by stimulating pH receptors.

All conditions that impair the ability of the lungs or chest wall to expand during inspiration cause dyspnea by triggering J, or stretch, receptors. Such conditions include airway obstructive disease, restrictive disease, and neuromuscular disorders.

Central nervous system–mediated dyspnea is uncommon. The prime example would be hyperventilation syndrome in which anxiety leads to triggering the respiratory center and to the sensation of dyspnea. On very rare occasions other central nervous system disorders can result in dyspnea. An example is given in the following clinical vignette.

CLINICAL VIGNETTE

One evening several years ago, a patient with AIDS was admitted to my service because of dyspnea. The patient had been hospitalized about 10 days earlier for the same complaint. At that time, the physical examination, the chest radiograph, and the arterial blood gases were totally normal. Despite those findings he was treated with intravenous pentamidine for presumed *Pneumocystis carinii* pneumonia. His dyspnea may have improved somewhat, and he was discharged—only to return several days later with the same complaint. The medical student admitting the patient again found a comfortable patient complaining of dyspnea; the physical examination, chest radiograph, and arterial blood gases were normal.

Because the student understood the mechanisms of dyspnea, she reasoned that acidosis could not be responsible—the patient's pH was normal. Nor was there any evidence to suggest a lung or chest wall problem that would trigger J receptors. She, therefore, focused on the possibility of a centrally mediated cause of the patient's dyspnea. She reviewed his medications and found that 10 days before the onset of dyspnea the patient had begun taking megestrol for anorexia. She consulted the literature and found that megestrol is a congener of progesterone, a drug sometimes used to treat central hypoventilation by directly triggering the respiratory center. She reasoned that megestrol might be responsible for the patient's dyspnea and discontinued the drug. The patient's dyspnea resolved and he was discharged.

22

Hypoxemia

There are five mechanisms by which hypoxemia may occur: low oxygen tension in inspired air, hypoventilation, low ventilation/perfusion ($\dot{V}/\dot{Q}$), decreased diffusion from the alveolus to the pulmonary capillary, and a right-to-left shunt. The first two causes are immediately apparent and cause no diagnostic dilemma, so the physician must generally distinguish among the latter three.

Conditions that result in the perfusion of areas that are not well ventilated are usually apparent by the patient's history and the physical examination. These disorders are usually characterized by bronchospasm or consolidation. Thus, the most difficult distinction is between disorders that cause a diffusion defect and those that cause a shunt. Examples of disorders causing a diffusion defect are pulmonary edema, other interstitial pulmonary infiltrates, sarcoidosis, and a number of fibrosing interstitial diseases. Right-to-left shunts may occur as a result of intracardiac defects, connections between the great vessels, pulmonary arteriovenous (AV) malformations, and the opening of numerous small AV shunts that bypass individual alveoli.

One example of the latter is pulmonary thromboembolism (PTE). Obstructing a pulmonary artery, even the right or left main pulmonary artery, with a clot does not in itself lead to hypoxemia, but rather simply leads to wasted ventilation. The area of the lung that is not perfused is still ventilated even though that ventilation is ineffective. However,

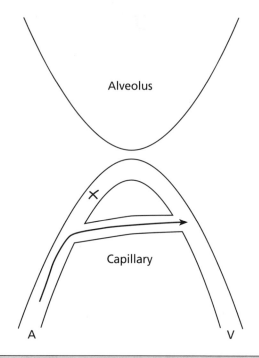

FIGURE 22.1
Shunting of Blood Through Small AV Shunts in PTE

PTEs may result in profound hypoxemia that is very difficult to correct with supplemental oxygen. The pathogenesis of hypoxemia in PTE is that the clot in the artery causes elaboration of mediators that cause profound vasodilation throughout the lungs, resulting in shunting of blood through small potential, but now open, AV shunts. Numerous alveoli that are ventilated are therefore not perfused, as demonstrated in Figure 22.1. A similar condition occurs in hepatopulmonary syndrome, in which a mediator causes similar vasodilation and the opening of potential AV shunts.

23

Shock

The circulatory system is a closed system containing fluid and a pump. Shock may occur as a consequence of one of three disorders. There may be a problem with the pump, there may be too little fluid in the system, or the amount of space in the system may be too great. Usually the cause of shock is fairly apparent. The chief distinction one needs to make is between a problem with the pump and a problem with either volume or space. If the pump is the culprit, then attention needs to be directed toward improving its function. For example, if there is something pressing on the pump, as in pericardial tamponade, or if there is a lesion that can be corrected surgically, such as valvular insufficiency or stenosis, those conditions need to be rectified.

Examples of shock due to too little volume in the circulation include hemorrhagic shock, external volume losses from sweating or diarrhea, and deposition of fluid into a third space, as occurs in intra-abdominal or retroperitoneal inflammatory processes such as severe pancreatitis. The most frequent cause of shock by virtue of expansion of the intravascular space is septic shock.

The treatment of shock caused by either too much space or too little volume is volume replacement. Volume should be pushed until the pulmonary capillary wedge pressure is at the high end of normal, regardless of any other physical finding or feature. For example, even if a patient in shock has edema for whatever reason, if the pulmonary capillary wedge pressure is low, then volume should be pushed vigorously. Pressors should be viewed only as very temporary, stopgap, life-saving measures for shock victims. They should be employed only to give one sufficient time to replace volume when shock is severe. One of the most common mistakes I have seen physicians make when they are treating shock is relying on pressors rather than pushing volume sufficiently.

24

Syncope and
Near Syncope

Evaluating syncope requires a very careful, clear, detailed patient history, because elucidating the cause of this symptom is usually accomplished through the history or not at all. Some causes of syncope are obvious, such as a blow to the head with a blunt object. The diagnostically challenging cases of syncope usually manifest as transient, self-limited events, in which the episode usually lasts only a few seconds or a few minutes. The events of the 1 to 2 seconds before the patient loses consciousness provide the most important clues to the mechanism of the syncope and thus to its cause.

There are three mechanisms by which transient loss of consciousness may occur: global hypoperfusion of the brain, hypoperfusion of the brain stem affecting the reticular activating system, and a seizure. Seizures are easy to diagnose when there is a witness who can describe tonic-clonic activity. When there is no such witness, historical and physical features such as the presence of an aura, a post-ictal state, tongue lacerations, extremely sore muscles, and evidence of bowel or bladder incontinence provide useful clues.

Historical features that point to syncope as having occurred by hypoperfusion of the brain stem include transient quadriparesis, ataxia or vertigo, and impairment of cranial nerve function, chiefly manifest as diplopia.

When seizure and vertebral-basilar insufficiency can be reasonably excluded, as is the case in most patients who present with syncope, we are left with global hypoperfusion of the brain. There are three mechanisms by which global hypoperfusion of the brain may occur transiently: a primary cardiac disorder, usually an arrhythmia but occasionally diminished cardiac output from a lesion such as aortic valvular stenosis; a vasovagal reaction; and a mismatch between intravascular volume and intravascular space such that the intravascular volume is too low or the intravascular space too large.

Historical features that suggest an arrhythmia include palpitations and a dramatic change in pulse rate, either too fast or too slow, especially if that change was instantaneous in onset. A vasovagal reaction is suggested by the patient's noticing progressively severe bradycardia, especially if it occurred in conjunction with an event known to trigger vasovagal reactions such as fear, nausea, difficult defecation, difficult micturition, or maneuvers that put pressure on the carotid sinus. Intravascular volume–space mismatch is suggested by the presence of tachycardia and by the onset of symptoms upon the patient's assuming an upright posture, especially in conjunction with an event that results in blood loss or volume depletion, or an event such as fever that increases the intravascular space.

25

Pericardial Tamponade

Pericardial tamponade occurs when fluid in the pericardium or, less commonly, scarring of the pericardium compromises the ability of the heart to function, thereby decreasing cardiac output. The chief detrimental effect of tamponade is to impair cardiac filling, of both the left side and the right side of the heart. Because of diminished filling of the left ventricle, left-sided cardiac output will fall and the patient's blood pressure will be low. Because of compression of the right atrium and right ventricle, filling of the right side of the heart will be diminished and Kussmaul's sign will be present. Kussmaul's sign is reversal of the normal pattern of jugular venous distention with the respiratory cycle. To understand why this reversal occurs, it is first necessary to understand the mechanisms by which the jugular pulse normally decreases during inspiration.

By decreasing intrathoracic pressure, inspiration causes venous return through the inferior and superior vena cavae to increase. This effect alone would tend to elevate the jugular venous pulse during inspiration, not decrease it. However, the increased return of blood to the right heart is more than compensated for by the right ventricle's distensibility and ability to accommodate all of the blood, and by the opening of additional pulmonary capillaries during inspiration which results in decreased pulmonary arteriolar

71

pressure and, therefore, decreased pressure against which the right ventricle must contract. Because the right ventricle's distensibility and the pulmonary capillary bed's lower pressure more than offset the increase in venous return, the jugular venous pressure falls during inspiration. In pericardial tamponade the right ventricle is no longer distensible and is unable to accommodate the increased venous return. Therefore, one gets a paradoxical venous pulse, namely an increase in jugular venous pressure with inspiration.

Similar phenomena explain the so-called paradoxical arterial pulse, which is not really paradoxical at all. Normally the arterial pulse falls 5 to 10 mm with inspiration. That is because inspiration results in the opening of pulmonary capillary beds (as discussed above) and thus a slight decrease in pulmonary vascular pressure. Some blood therefore "pools" in the enlarged pulmonary vascular bed, resulting in slightly diminished return to the left atrium and left ventricle; this results in slightly diminished cardiac output during that phase of the respiratory cycle. In pericardial tamponade, the pulmonary vasculature open normally during inspiration, but the right ventricle is unable to increase its output and to fill the newly opened vascular beds. The result is even more pulmonary vascular "pooling" of blood, a marked decrease in left atrial and left ventricular filling, and a more marked drop in systemic blood pressure. These events are further compounded by the increased venous return during inspiration resulting in distensibility of the portion of the right ventricle that is not limited by the pericardial tamponade, namely the ventricular septum. The resulting septal bulge into the left ventricle further diminishes left ventricular filling, left ventricular output, and blood pressure.

26

Diastolic Runoff Physiology

Diastolic runoff is a situation in which blood can escape from the arterial tree during diastole. The differential diagnosis of runoff physiology is fairly narrow. The classic example is aortic valve regurgitation. However, the most common runoff situation is exercise, in which numerous capillary beds that were not open are now open. During diastole blood can "run off" into these newly opened capillary beds, thereby markedly lowering diastolic pressure. Anemia, fever, and thyrotoxicosis cause similar physiology. Other examples include systemic arteriovenous malformations or fistulae and patent ductus arteriosis, situations in which blood can run off from the systemic arterial circulation into much lower pressure vessels such as systemic veins or the pulmonary artery.

The signs of runoff physiology include very low diastolic blood pressure, and the plethora of findings of aortic valve regurgitation such as head bobbing, water hammer pulses, pistol shot femoral pulses, Hill's sign, and rapid rise and fall of the arterial pulse. These signs are for the most part due to a secondary phenomenon. When diastolic blood pressure is low, there is usually a reflex tachycardia and the circulation is "fast." Thus, ventricular filling is both rapid and greater than normal, and the ejection fraction is greater than normal, often resulting in sometimes markedly elevated systolic pressure. The findings we associate with, for example, aortic valve regurgitation are due to a combination of very rapid and very forceful left ventricular emptying followed by diastolic runoff resulting in collapse of the arterial pulse.

27

Atrial Septal Defect

Atrial septal defect is a cardiac lesion that may escape detection for decades because it often causes no symptoms and the signs are quite subtle. In atrial septal defect some of the blood returning to the left atrium passes through the defect into the right atrium; thus, the physiology is right-sided circulatory volume overload. The signs include fixed splitting of the second heart sound and a soft systolic ejection murmur over the pulmonary outflow tract. No murmur occurs as a result of blood going from the left atrium to the right atrium because there is an insufficient pressure gradient between those two chambers to generate a murmur. Because the atrial septal defect persists for decades, later signs may include a right ventricular lift or bulge and eventually signs of cor pulmonale.

It is important that the physician detect the early telltale signs of atrial septal defect so that it can be repaired before irreversible damage is done. Normally the second heart sound split widens during inspiration because the negative intrathoracic pressure generated by inspiration leads to an increase in venous return and in the volume of blood delivered to the right ventricle and subsequently to an increase in right ventricular output. When the right ventricle pumps that much blood, it takes longer to empty, thereby delaying closure of the pulmonic valve and exaggerating the split of the second heart sound. In patients with atrial septal defect there is constantly excessive blood being delivered to the right ventricle. Therefore, there will not be a respiratory change in the split of the second heart sound, but rather a persistent split. The soft systolic pulmonary outflow murmur is simply a flow murmur generated because of the high volume being delivered across the pulmonary outflow tract.

PART IV

HEMATOLOGIC DISORDERS

28

Coombs' Tests

I have found that most students and house officers have a fairly poor understanding of how Coombs' tests are performed or how to interpret the results.

The direct Coombs' test is performed by incubating the patient's erythrocytes with an antibody directed against human IgG and human C3. After an appropriate incubation period, microscopic agglutination is sought. Erythrocyte agglutination indicates a positive test, non-agglutination a negative test. Another name for the direct Coombs' test is the DAT (direct antiglobulin test).

The indirect Coombs' test is performed by incubating a panel of erythrocytes first with the patient's serum and then with antibody to human IgG. Again microscopic agglutination indicates a positive test, non-agglutination a negative test. Another name for the indirect Coombs' test is the antibody screen.

Proper interpretation of the results of these tests should focus not on where the antibody is (i.e., on the patient's erythrocytes or in the patient's serum), but rather on the immunologic specificity of the antibody. There are four possible results of the Coombs' tests (Table 28.1). Both tests can be negative, which is normal.

A positive indirect Coombs' test with a negative direct Coombs' test indicates that a patient has antibodies in the serum that react with somebody else's erythrocytes but not his or her own. Almost always these antibodies are directed

TABLE 28.1
Interpretation of Coombs' Test Results

Coombs' Test		Interpretation
Direct	Indirect	
−	−	Normal
−	+	Alloantibody
+	+	Autoantibody
+	−	Drug-induced or autoantibody

against blood group antigens and are the result of prior transfusion or multiparity. The blood bank will usually not only report that the indirect Coombs' test, or the antibody screen, is positive but will also report the identity of the antibody contained in the patient's serum.

A positive direct Coombs' test and positive indirect Coombs' test means that the patient has an antibody that reacts with both his or her own erythrocytes and those of others—almost certainly an autoantibody that reacts with intrinsic erythrocyte protein(s), not with blood group antigens.

The situation that provides the greatest difficulty in interpretation is a positive direct Coombs' test in the face of a negative indirect Coombs' test. Here there are two possibilities. First, the antibody on the patient's erythrocytes may be directed not toward an erythrocyte component but rather toward a drug coating the erythrocyte. Penicillin-induced hemolytic anemia is the classic example of such a finding. Alternatively, the patient may have an autoantibody that has such a high affinity and is present in such low concentration in the serum that essentially all of it is on the patient's erythrocytes. The quantity in the serum is so low that it is insufficient to coat erythrocytes used in the indirect test.

When the direct Coombs' test is positive, the blood bank personnel will elute the antibody from the erythrocyte by dropping the pH of the suspension (which breaks antigen–antibody bonds), centrifuging the erythrocytes, recovering the supernatant containing the antibody, and restoring the pH to physiologic. They will then incubate this eluate with a panel of erythrocytes in an attempt to determine the identity of the antibody. If the antibody is an autoantibody, as is usually the case, it will react with all the erythrocytes tested; the laboratory will not be able to determine the identity of the antibody and will report this to the physician. The physician should conclude that the patient has an autoantibody.

Finally, when the direct Coombs' test is positive when a mixture of antibody directed against human IgG and antibody against human C3 is used, the blood bank personnel will then use selective antibodies directed against either IgG or C3 to identify which molecule is present on the patient's erythrocytes. Most of the time the molecule is IgG, and the discussion in the preceding paragraphs applies. Occasionally the molecule is C3. When C3, but not IgG, is present on the erythrocyte, it usually means that the patient has a cold IgM autoantibody. These antibodies undergo a conformational change at temperatures slightly below 37°C, temperatures that are common in the distal circulation such as that in the limbs. The conformational change results in the antibody recognizing a component on the erythrocyte, binding to the erythrocyte, and fixing complement onto its surface. As the erythrocyte returns to the more proximal circulation and rewarms, the IgM autoantibody reverses its conformational change and falls off the erythrocyte, leaving only C3 covalently bound. Thus, the presence of C3 on the erythrocyte usually indicates the presence of a cold IgM autoantibody. This antibody can be sought specifically by obtaining plasma under conditions of warmth and cooling it in the laboratory to allow the IgM to bind to erythrocytes.

CLINICAL VIGNETTE

A 40-year-old man was hospitalized for disseminated histoplasmosis, which had relapsed after treatment with amphotericin B followed by itraconazole for several months. Because he was severely anemic, an antibody screen (indirect Coombs' test) was performed in the course of typing and cross-matching his blood in anticipation of transfusion. The laboratory reported that the antibody screen was positive but that they were unable to identify the antibody. Realizing that the laboratory's inability to identify the antibody meant that the antibody reacted with their entire panel of erythrocytes and that the patient probably had an autoantibody, the house-staff ordered a direct antiglobulin test (direct Coombs' test). It was likewise positive, and the eluate reacted with all erythrocytes tested by the blood bank personnel. The house-staff was puzzled as to why the patient should have an autoantibody, because disseminated histoplasmosis should not cause such a problem. So they began a search for an underlying disease that could be responsible not only for rendering the patient unusually susceptible to histoplasmosis, but also for producing an autoantibody. A bone marrow biopsy revealed lymphoma.

In this case, knowledge that a positive antibody screen with an antibody not directed against a blood group antigen likely meant that the antibody was an autoantibody led the house-staff to seek confirmation with a direct antiglobulin test. The test findings then led to a search for, and the identification of, an illness other than the one with which the patient had presented that would explain both his autoantibody and his infectious disease.

29

Hemolytic Anemia

Hemolysis may occur by many mechanisms (Table 29.1).

One mechanism of hemolysis is the plasma membrane being damaged directly and selectively. In clostridial infections, for example, lecithinase elaborated by the microorganism destroys lecithin in the erythrocyte plasma membrane and leads to hemolysis. In paroxysmal nocturnal hemoglobinuria, the proteins that normally protect the erythrocyte against the lytic action of complement are missing; therefore, erythrocytes are lysed by even the low levels of activated complement that are produced day in and day out. Finally, in autoimmune hemolytic anemia, IgG antibody binds to the erythrocyte surface. Here the mechanism of destruction is not usually complement-mediated but rather phagocytosis via splenic macrophages which recognize the Fc portion of IgG via their Fc receptors.

A second mechanism of hemolysis is a defect in an important structural protein such as ankyrin or spectrin, as occurs in congenital spherocytosis or elliptocytosis. Disorders of hemoglobin are a third cause of hemolysis. Sickle cell disease as well as thalassemia, for example, causes important structural changes in either the hemoglobin molecule itself or the globin chains with important implications for friability of the erythrocytes. Fourth, infection of the erythrocyte with certain microorganisms renders it friable and actually lyses it. Examples include bartonellosis, malaria, and babesiosis. Fifth, the absence of an enzyme to

TABLE 29.1
Mechanisms and Causes of Hemolytic Anemia

Erythrocytic Plasma Membrane Damage
Lecithinase from *Clostridia*
Paroxysmal nocturnal hemoglobinuria
Autoimmune hemolytic anemia

Intra-Erythrocytic Disorder
Defective structural protein
Defective hemoglobin
Intra-erythrocytic infection
    Bartonellosis
    Malaria
    Babesiosis
G-6-PD deficiency
Pernicious anemia

Extra-Erythrocytic Disorder
Hypersplenism
Disseminated intravascular coagulation
TTP-HUS
Prosthetic heart valve

metabolize reactive oxygen metabolites, as seen in glucose 6-phosphate dehydrogenase (G-6-PD) deficiency, results in hemolysis when greater than normal quantities of oxidative metabolites are produced, such as with primaquine administration. Sixth, erythrocytes that are manufactured with deficiencies of certain important components such as vitamin B_{12} are very friable and have a markedly shortened half-life in the circulation. Sometimes, they are so friable that their rate of destruction actually results in hemolytic anemia.

Finally, events outside the erythrocyte itself but within the vascular system may have important implications for the survival of erythrocytes. For example, the spleen's enlargement for any reason enables the numerous splenic macrophages to phagocytize erythrocytes. Disseminated intravascular coagulation entangles erythrocytes in clots and destroys them. Disorders of the microcirculation itself such as thrombotic thrombocytopenic purpura (TTP)/hemolytic uremic syndrome (HUS) result in the physical destruction of erythrocytes intravascularly. Damage to erythrocytes by devices such as prosthetic heart valves can also cause hemolysis.

Laboratory findings in hemolytic anemia include an elevated level of lactate dehydrogenase (LDH), which is released from erythrocytes as they are lysed, and an elevated level of indirect bilirubin because the liver is unable to process the large quantities of hemoglobin metabolic products presented to it as a result of hemolysis. Serum haptoglobin is a protein that binds hemoglobin; its value will usually fall to zero and there will be free hemoglobin present in the serum in hemolytic anemia. If the bone marrow is able, it will respond to anemia with reticulocytosis, and reticulocytosis is a secondary sign of hemolytic anemia. Finally, if one is suspicious that hemolysis may have occurred within the preceding week but the signs and laboratory features of active hemolysis are not currently present, hemosiderin will continue to be excreted in the urine for up to one week after a hemolytic event and can be sought to develop evidence for hemolysis.

30

Large Erythrocytes

There are two basic mechanisms by which large erythrocytes are present in the circulation. The first is reticulocytosis; reticulocytes are larger than mature erythrocytes. The second and most common mechanism is interference with DNA metabolism in the developing erythrocyte. When DNA synthesis is impaired, the erythrocyte's cytoplasm matures but the nucleus cannot, resulting in nuclear–cytoplasmic dissociation and an erythrocyte whose cytoplasmic compartment grows for a prolonged period before the nucleus matures and is ejected. Lack of folic acid and lack of vitamin B_{12} are the classic causes of anemia with large erythrocytes. Drugs used to treat HIV infection that interfere with DNA replication of the virus also interfere with DNA replication by the erythrocyte, so most patients on antiretroviral therapy will have very large erythrocytes. Alcoholism and chronic liver disease cause large erythrocytes as well, probably by impairing DNA synthesis.

31

Eosinophilia

Eosinophilia may occur by three major mechanisms: the release of eosinophil chemotactic factor of anaphylaxis (ECF-A) from mast cells, the elaboration of interleukin-5 (IL-5 or eosinophilopoietin) from helper T cells, and a disorder of myelopoiesis such as eosinophilic leukemia (Table 31.1). When mast cells are degranulated—for example, by bridging two IgE molecules on their surfaces—ECF-A is released from the granule in addition to histamine and other mediators. It attracts eosinophils to the site. Thus, Type I hypersensitivity is associated with eosinophilia. A second mechanism by which mast cells may be degranulated is by engagement of their cell surface receptors for C3a, the small fragment of cleaved C3 also known as anaphylatoxin. Types II and III hypersensitivity result in complement activation, cleavage of C3, binding of C3a to mast cell receptors, degranulation of the mast cell, release of ECF-A, and therefore eosinophilia. Immunologically mediated mast cell degranulation is called anaphylaxis. Certain drugs, such as vancomycin, morphine, and contrast dye, directly bind to and degranulate mast cells, a condition known as an anaphylactoid reaction. Finally, the disease mastocytosis causes spontaneous degranulation of mast cells with release of ECF-A and eosinophilia.

The major recognized promoter of eosinophil development and release from the bone marrow is IL-5, produced by helper T cells. IL-5 is produced by and released from

TABLE 31.1
Mechanisms and Causes of Eosinophilia

Release of ECF-A by Mast Cells	*Interleukin 5 from T Lymphocytes*
Type I hypersensitivity	Migrating helminth larvae
C3a	HIV infection
Type II hypersensitivity	Hodgkin's disease/Lymphoma
Type III hypersensitivity	Hypereosinophilic syndromes
Drugs	Adrenal insufficiency
Vancomycin	*Disordered Myelopoiesis*
Morphine	Eosinophilic leukemia
Contrast dye	Myelofibrosis with myeloid
Mastocytosis	metaplasia

these cells when their surface receptors are engaged by products of migrating helminthic larvae. It is also released when the gene is turned on by HIV infection or when the cells become malignant, as in lymphoma. The various hypereosinophilic syndromes, including eosinophilic cardiomyopathy and eosinophilic gastroenteritis, are disorders in which there is overproduction of IL-5, resulting in very high eosinophil counts and in some cases invasion of and damage to specific organs. Lymphocytes are regulated in part by endogenous corticosteroids, which downregulate most of their functions. When corticosteroids are deficient, as in adrenal insufficiency, the normally suppressive effect of these molecules is absent and lymphocytes overproduce some cytokines including IL-5, often resulting in moderate eosinophilia.

Examples of disordered myelopoiesis that results in eosinophilia include eosinophilic leukemia and myelofibrosis with myeloid metaplasia.

CLINICAL VIGNETTE

A 40-year-old man presented with a 6-month history of progressively severe weakness, easy fatigability, and low-grade fever. He had been able to continue his work as an accountant, but for the past month he had been barely able to complete his day's work and was too exhausted to do anything but eat dinner and retire to bed after work. The physical examination was unremarkable. The laboratory examination was likewise unremarkable except for the finding of 12% eosinophils in the peripheral blood. The bone marrow examination revealed only somewhat elevated numbers of eosinophils. His HIV antibody titer was negative. CT scans of the chest and abdomen were normal.

The house-staff reasoned that mast cell degranulation and myeloproliferative disease were not the mechanism of the patient's eosinophilia, so they focused on diseases associated with increased IL-5. Larval migration would not likely cause fever and constitutional symptoms for months, and lymphoma seemed unlikely in light of the bone marrow and CT scan results. The house-staff obtained serum cortisol levels before and after administration of Cortrosyn and found them to be very low. The patient's symptoms resolved when he was treated with replacement cortisol.

In this case, careful reasoning enabled the house-staff to make a diagnosis of a very unusual cause of chronic fever and eosinophilia. When corticosteroids are deficient, unsuppressed production of IL-1 and IL-5 can cause fever and eosinophilia, respectively.

32

Thrombocytopenia

Thrombocytopenia occurs either as the result of diminished platelet production by the bone marrow or increased platelet destruction peripherally. There are numerous causes of diminished platelet production, including diseases such as leukemia, primary bone marrow failure, deficiency of important nutritional factors such as vitamin B_{12}, toxic or idiosyncratic reactions to drugs, and replacement of the marrow by an infectious agent or a neoplasm. The mechanisms responsible for peripheral platelet destruction include complement-mediated destruction in paroxysmal nocturnal hemoglobinuria, hypersplenism, disseminated intravascular coagulation, TTP-HUS, and antibody-mediated destruction.

There are two major mechanisms by which immunologically mediated destruction of platelets may occur. The first is autoimmune, i.e., the patient generates an antibody that recognizes a molecule on the platelet surface, binds to it and opsonizes the platelet for rapid ingestion by splenic macrophages. This is the mechanism of injury in idiopathic thrombocytopenic purpura (ITP) and in heparin-induced thrombocytopenia. More commonly platelets are injured by immune complexes. Like most leukocytes, platelets have on their surfaces receptors for the Fc portion of IgG. Circulating immune complexes bind to these receptors and damage platelets by two mechanisms. First, the binding to and bridging of platelet Fc receptors causes them to degranulate. Second, platelets with immune complexes bound to their surfaces are opsonized and readily recognized by Fc receptors on the surfaces of macrophages, which ingest and destroy them.

One can distinguish readily between the two primary mechanisms of thrombocytopenia, diminished production and peripheral destruction, by obtaining a bone marrow sample and looking for megakaryocytes. They will be deficient in the first case and more than plentiful in the second. Once one has determined either by bone marrow examination or by the clinical setting that peripheral destruction is the mechanism responsible for a patient's thrombocytopenia, a very useful test is to determine platelet-associated antibodies. These will be increased in number in immune-mediated thrombocytopenia whether autoimmune or immune complex in nature. Initial urgent treatment of immune-mediated thrombocytopenia is directed toward blocking the macrophages', and in immune complex disease blocking the platelets', Fc receptors either by overloading them with monovalent antibody by the intravenous administration of immunoglobulin or by markedly diminishing the affinity of the cells' Fc receptors for the Fc portion of IgG by the administration of corticosteroids.

CLINICAL VIGNETTE

A 35-year-old man presented after several months of progressively severe malaise. The physical examination was normal. The complete blood cell count revealed pancytopenia with a WBC count of 2500/μL, a packed cell volume of 28%, and a platelet count of 35,000/μL. The bone marrow was slightly hypocellular but contained greater than normal numbers of megakaryocytes. Because the mechanism of thrombocytopenia seemed likely to be peripheral platelet destruction, the house-staff obtained platelet-associated antibodies. They were strikingly elevated.

The fact that the patient had pancytopenia rather than only thrombocytopenia suggested a more generalized illness than ITP, and suggested that the patient had platelet-bound immune complexes rather than an antiplatelet antibody. There was no evidence for lymphoma or primary immunologic disease such as systemic lupus erythematosus, and the antinuclear antibody titer was negative. The house-staff obtained an HIV antibody; it was positive.

With this patient, HIV infection presented with pancytopenia rather than with an opportunistic infection. Focusing on the thrombocytopenia enabled the house-staff first to define the mechanism of thrombocytopenia and then to identify the specific cause by thoroughly reasoning through the possible causes of immune complex disease.

33

Thrombocytosis

There are two major mechanisms by which platelet elevation may occur: an abnormality of megakaryocyte regulation in the bone marrow and chronic inflammation. During
chronic inflammatory states, macrophages are triggered to
produce a molecule, thrombopoietin, that causes megakaryocytes to overproduce platelets. In these conditions
thrombocytosis is usually in the range of 500,000 to 1
million/μL.

Examples of thrombocytosis caused by abnormal regulation of megakaryocytes include megakaryocytic leukemia
and polycythemia rubra vera (PRV). In these conditions,
platelet counts are usually over 1 million/μL.

Thrombocytosis due to chronic inflammatory states is
much more common than thrombocytosis caused by a primary bone marrow disorder. Unless a chronic inflammatory
condition is apparent, it may be difficult to distinguish
between the two mechanisms. However, a few ancillary
studies may help. For example, in chronic inflammatory conditions sufficient to cause thrombocytosis, the erythrocyte
sedimentation rate is usually quite elevated. Anemia of
chronic disease is generally present in chronic inflammatory
disorders, whereas erythrocytosis is present in PRV. The WBC
count is often elevated in both conditions and is not diagnostically useful, but determining the level of leukocyte
alkaline phosphatase may be especially helpful because it is
elevated in PRV but normal in chronic inflammatory disorders.

Finally, although bone marrow examination will usually reveal numerous megakaryocytes in both conditions, it may reveal other abnormalities when the cause is a disorder of megakaryocyte regulation.

In addition to these two major mechanisms, several others are occasionally encountered. Patients who have had a splenectomy commonly have somewhat elevated platelet counts simply because the spleen normally removes some platelets from the circulation. A second mechanism is elaboration of large quantities of erythropoietin, which is structurally similar to thrombopoietin and has stimulatory effects on megakaryocytes. Iron deficiency anemia and chronic hemolytic anemias are common causes of elaboration of erythropoietin and are associated with moderate thrombocytosis. Finally, rebound thrombocytosis occurs after recovery from conditions of bone marrow suppression. Presumably the mechanism here is the effect of large quantities of thrombopoietin on megakaryocytes that were formerly unable to respond to the molecule. When no other cause for thrombocytosis can be identified, the condition is referred to as essential thrombocytosis.

CLINICAL VIGNETTE

An 85-year-old woman was hospitalized because of sepsis. She was a nursing home resident who was severely demented and bedbound. She had grade 2 sacral and hip decubitus ulcers and a chronic Foley catheter. Each of the prior 3 months she had been admitted for a similar condition. Blood and urine cultures had each grown enteric gram-negative rods; this time blood grew *Klebsiella* and the urine grew *Klebsiella* and *Escherichia coli*. She had been treated with appropriate antibiotics for a urinary tract infection with sepsis on each of the prior admissions. When the fever and signs of sepsis resolved, she was discharged—only to return within 2 weeks with an identical illness.

When her platelet count was found to be 750,000/µL on the current admission, as it had been on two prior admissions, the house-staff reasoned that a recurrent urinary tract infection was not likely responsible for her repeated illnesses, but rather it might be a chronic inflammatory process. Even though the decubitus ulcers did not seem deep, the house-staff obtained a CT scan of her pelvis. It revealed a large abscess contiguous with one of the ulcers. The abscess was drained, and after an appropriate duration of antimicrobial therapy the patient was discharged to the nursing home.

It is impossible to know with certainty that a urinary tract infection is responsible for a febrile illness or even bacteremia in a patient who has an indwelling Foley catheter. Growing the same bacterium from blood and urine is suggestive, but urine from patients with indwelling catheters will nearly always grow a gram-negative rod even when the patient is not ill; gram-negative rod bacteremia may be related to an infection elsewhere, not a urinary tract infection. In this case, the house-staff recognized that thrombocytosis strongly suggested a chronic inflammatory process, which led them to search for, and to find, a pelvic abscess. It was the pelvic abscess, not urinary tract infection, that had been responsible for the patient's prior episodes of sepsis. Because the abscess had not been identified and drained, the first three episodes responded transiently to antibiotic treatment only to relapse after the antibiotics were stopped.

34

Leukemoid Reaction

A leukemoid reaction is leukocytosis with a left shift containing band forms, metamyelocytes, myelocytes, and occasionally even a few blasts. Generally the number of neutrophils is greater than the number of band forms, which is greater than the number of metamyelocytes, which is greater than the number of myelocytes. There are two fundamental mechanisms by which a leukemoid reaction may occur: a disorder of regulation of the development of neutrophils in the bone marrow or the elaboration of a molecule such as G-CSF which influences the development of neutrophils. The usual differential diagnosis is among chronic myelogenous leukemia (CML), PRV, and a secondary leukemoid reaction. The single most useful test to distinguish among these is the leukocyte alkaline phosphatase (LAP) determination. It will be elevated in PRV, normal in secondary leukemoid reactions, and depressed in granulocytic leukemia.

Diseases associated with secondary leukemoid reactions (elevated levels of G-CSF) include miliary tuberculosis, abscesses, and a marrow recovering from suppression. In the latter case, presumably the granulocyte progenitors' receptors are saturated with G-CSF, which has been bound to them while they were unable to respond. Now that they are able to respond, they do so with a vengeance.

CLINICAL VIGNETTE

A 60-year-old man presented with a history of several months of progressively severe fatigue, a 25-pound weight loss, and a low-grade fever. The physical examination was unremarkable except for the signs of weight loss. The laboratory evaluation revealed signs of chronic disease, anemia and hypoalbuminemia, and a white blood cell count of 25,000/μL with 50% neutrophils, 20% band forms, 10% metamyelocytes, and 5% myelocytes. The LAP score was normal. The house-staff reasoned that the absence of erythrocytosis and thrombocytosis as well as the normal LAP score made PRV very unlikely. CML seemed unlikely because the LAP score was not low. The most likely diagnosis appeared to be a chronic infectious disorder. When the CT scan of the abdomen failed to reveal an occult intra-abdominal abscess, the house-staff placed a tuberculin skin test. It reacted with 25 mm of induration. They began antituberculous therapy empirically. The patient improved within 2 weeks. Four weeks later *Mycobacterium tuberculosis* grew from a bone marrow sample that had been obtained during the initial evaluation.

The evaluation of the leukemoid reaction with a LAP score, combined with other signs that made PRV and CML less likely, led the house-staff to pursue an infectious cause. Careful and thorough evaluation led to the presumptive, and later the definitive, diagnosis of miliary tuberculosis.

PART V

GASTROINTESTINAL AND HEPATIC DISORDERS

35

Liver Function Tests

The vast array of liver function tests available sometimes leads to confusion over the pathophysiologic significance of an abnormality in each test. I focus on the results of only four determinations because each determination provides specific information about the nature of the liver injury and gives information different from the other three.

An elevation in the AST means there has been hepatocellular necrosis. AST, like LDH, is a cytoplasmic enzyme that is released upon cell death.

Prolongation of the prothrombin time indicates that more than 95% of hepatocytes have been destroyed because 5% of functioning hepatocytes is sufficient to produce adequate quantities of coagulation factors.

Elevation of bilirubin may occur by two hepatic mechanisms: obstruction of the common bile duct, or a biochemical defect in the ability of the liver to conjugate or to secrete bilirubin. Examples of the latter include Gilbert's disease and Criegler-Najjar abnormality, congenital disorders in the liver's ability to handle bilirubin. However, the most common cause of hyperbilirubinemia by this mechanism is sick hepatocytes. Examples include inability of hepatocytes that are injured but not killed by hepatitis viruses to conjugate and secrete bilirubin during the course of acute viral hepatitis and "poisoning" of the hepatocyte by as yet undetermined molecules in a number of systemic diseases such as pneumococcal infection.

Alkaline phosphatase is secreted by hepatocytes lining biliary ductules when those cells are subjected to pressure. Pressure may come from the duct side, such as when the common bile duct is obstructed; or pressure may come from the other side, such as when there is a mass lesion in the liver exerting pressure on those cells. The mass lesion or lesions may be large and may therefore be seen on CT scan or ultrasound, or they may be small but numerous, such as in disseminated infection with *Mycobacterium avium* complex in AIDS, for example. In the latter case, the alkaline phosphatase may be 8 or 10 times normal, but ultrasound and CT scan will fail to reveal space-occupying lesions because each lesion is too small to be seen by those techniques. However, the lesions are sufficiently numerous to exert pressure on many hepatocytes, triggering them to elaborate alkaline phosphatase.

I find that by understanding these mechanisms of hepatocyte injury and response to injury, I am better able to focus on the appropriate differential diagnosis and to more expeditiously make a specific diagnosis. For example, in a patient whose dominant hepatic dysfunction is a very high AST, I would initially order serologies for hepatitis viruses. In contrast, in a patient whose dominant hepatic dysfunction is a markedly elevated alkaline phosphatase, I would order an imaging study of the liver.

CLINICAL VIGNETTE

A 30-year-old man with late-stage HIV infection was found to have an alkaline phosphatase level of 1100 U/L and a γ-glutamyltransferase (GGT) level of 1000 U/L. Except for moderate fatigue, he had no symptoms and the remaining liver function tests were normal. The house-staff reasoned that the cause of his hepatic dysfunction was either common bile duct obstruction or intrahepatic mass lesion. An ultrasound study of the abdomen failed to reveal either dilated bile ducts or a hepatic lesion. They then reasoned that the pathogenesis of his elevated alkaline phosphatase was likely multiple small space-occupying hepatic lesions that were pressing on ductile hepatocytes and causing them to make alkaline phosphatase. A disseminated opportunistic infection seemed likely. Rather than biopsying either the liver or the bone marrow, the house-staff initially obtained blood cultures for mycobacteria and fungi. *Mycobacterium avium* complex grew from the blood, and they began the appropriate antimycobacterial therapy.

For this patient, the pattern of hepatic dysfunction led the house-staff not to pursue studies for hepatitis or other causes of hepatic injury, but rather to focus on extrahepatic bile duct obstruction or intrahepatic space occupying lesions. When neither obstruction nor a large hepatic mass was identified, they sought a cause of multiple space-occupying intrahepatic lesions and initially performed the least invasive study to identify such a cause. They were rewarded when the blood cultures were positive.

36

Diarrhea

The pathogenesis of diarrhea depends upon whether the cause of diarrhea is located in the small bowel or the large bowel. Small bowel–mediated diarrhea is caused either by secretion of fluid by the gut epithelial cells or by a molecule or molecules in the gut lumen that exert osmotic pressure and are responsible for delivering both themselves and large volumes of water to the large bowel. The absorptive capacity of the large bowel is quite limited. The colon normally absorbs a little less than a liter of fluid a day and is capable of absorbing only a few liters a day. Therefore, any volume greater than a few liters that is delivered to the ileocecal valve will pass through the colon and result in diarrhea.

The major causes of secretory diarrhea are infectious agents such as *Vibrio cholerae* and molecules such as vasoactive intestinal peptide which cause gut epithelial cells to secrete. Osmotic molecules include lactose, a cause of diarrhea in those with lactase deficiency; glucose, in those with dumping syndrome; small molecules contained in certain laxatives; bile salts; and, most commonly, small molecules such as amino acids and sugars derived from digested food that cannot be absorbed in certain diseases of the small bowel epithelia or the lamina propria. Examples of disorders of the gut epithelium include sprue, which denudes the epithelia, and certain protozoal infections, which populate the epithelia cells and prevent absorption of small molecules derived from digested food. Examples of diseases of the lamina propria include lymphoma and amyloidosis, which infiltrate the lamina propria and interfere with the ability of digested food products to be absorbed properly.

Distinguishing between secretory and absorptive diarrhea is accomplished in two ways. One can measure stool electrolytes and osmolality and simultaneously calculate the osmolality that is attributable to electrolytes. A gap between measured and calculated osmolality of 100 mOsm/L or more is strongly suggestive of osmotic diarrhea. In secretory diarrhea the gap is much narrower. The second way to distinguish is to have the patient fast: secretory diarrhea should continue, whereas osmotic diarrhea should stop because no osmotically active molecules should be present in the gut lumen.

Understanding the pathogenesis of small bowel diarrhea allows us to predict the signs and symptoms and some laboratory findings. For example, the patient will not usually have fever, and abdominal pain (if any) should be minimal with only occasional periumbilical cramping. Because the stimulus to defecate is the presence of large volumes of water in the rectum, each trip to the toilet should be quite productive and the diarrhea should be predominantly water. The frequency of diarrhea will depend on the volume of water presented to the rectum, and it may range from a few times a day to very many times a day. Finally, as the process is not inflammatory, there should be no leukocytes in the stool.

The pathogenesis of large bowel–mediated diarrhea is usually inflammation. The symptoms and signs should include fever, lower abdominal pain; tenesmus; rectal urgency; and the passage of blood, pus, and mucus in the stool. Because the stimulus to defecate is rectal irritation by inflammation, the patient may make numerous trips to the toilet but may produce only blood, pus, mucus, gas, small amounts of water, and small amounts of stool. Because inflammation is the cause of diarrhea, the stool should contain numerous leukocytes. Examples of inflammatory diarrhea include the bacterial causes of colitis, inflammatory bowel diseases, *Clostridium difficile* toxin-mediated colitis, diverticulitis, and in AIDS patients cytomegalovirus colitis.

Two noninflammatory colonic disorders may mimic small bowel–mediated diarrhea. So-called collagenous colitis impairs water absorption by the colon and thus causes moderate watery diarrhea. Rectal villous adenomas cause secretion of large quantities of water and electrolytes. These tumors are usually palpable on digital examination of the rectum.

In most cases the patient's history, the physical findings, and the determination of fecal leukocytes should allow us to rapidly determine whether the condition is in the small bowel or the large bowel and to focus our subsequent evaluation efficiently. For example, when the signs and symptoms suggest colitis and the stool contains numerous leukocytes, culturing the stool for enteric pathogens is appropriate. When the signs and symptoms and the absence of fecal leukocytes suggest a small bowel condition, then our initial efforts should be to determine whether diarrhea is secretory or osmotic. Occasionally one encounters a patient who has features of both; that is, the patient may have fever and constitutional symptoms and yet have high-volume, watery diarrhea without fecal leukocytes. Here the pathogenesis often is in the small bowel. For example, the patient may have viral gastroenteritis, in which the virus coats the gut epithelia and causes osmotic diarrhea while at the same time disseminating and causing constitutional symptoms including fever. Alternatively, the lamina propria may be infiltrated with an infectious agent that is causing osmotic diarrhea, such as *Mycobacterium avium* complex in AIDS patients. That same agent may also be disseminated and causing constitutional symptoms including fever. If the physician focuses clearly on the pathophysiologic mechanisms of diarrhea, these complicated problems can usually be reasoned through carefully and solved expeditiously.

CLINICAL VIGNETTE

A 30-year-old man with late-stage HIV infection presented with fever and diarrhea. Both had begun 10 days earlier. His fever had ranged from 100°F to 103°F (38° to 39°C), and the diarrhea was voluminous, watery, and frequent, averaging 6 to 12 stools a day. He denied tenesmus and had noted no blood, pus, or mucus in his stool. He had experienced only minimal periumbilical cramping. There were no leukocytes in the stool.

The house-staff reasoned that, whereas fever suggested an inflammatory, large bowel–mediated diarrhea, both his gastrointestinal symptoms and the absence of leukocytes from stool were more suggestive of a process mediated by the small bowel. They then considered that fever might indicate a systemic infectious illness and that the diarrhea was due to infiltration of the lamina propria by the same microbe responsible for the fever. They therefore obtained blood cultures for mycobacteria and fungi, and obtained cultures and special stains of the stool for mycobacteria. The stain of stool revealed acid-fast bacteria, and both cultures grew *Mycobacterium avium* complex.

This patient had presented with some signs and symptoms that suggested small bowel–mediated diarrhea, but others that suggested an inflammatory, large bowel–mediated diarrhea. The house-staff reasoned that the pathogenesis of the patient's diarrhea was likely small bowel–mediated and not an inflammatory process. Their focus on a disseminated infectious process that might cause fever as well as infiltration of the lamina propria leading to small bowel–mediated, watery diarrhea led them expeditiously to make the appropriate diagnosis.

37

Elevated Amylase Levels

Amylase is produced by salivary glands, pancreas, and fallopian tubes. The differential diagnosis of elevated levels of serum amylase thus includes disorders of these organs that disrupt their integrity and allow amylase to gain access to the bloodstream. The greatest concentrations of amylase are contained in the gastrointestinal tract. Disorders of the gastrointestinal tract that disrupt its integrity allow amylase access to the bloodstream. For example, amylase produced by the salivary glands is normally swallowed and may gain access to the bloodstream when esophageal disorders are present, most especially a ruptured esophagus. Likewise, disorders of the small bowel, most especially ischemia of the small bowel, may cause very high elevations of serum amylase. A stone in the common bile duct that obstructs the flow of pancreatic juice to the duodenum and diverts it retrograde up the common bile duct and into the liver may allow amylase entry to the bloodstream via the liver; so elevations of serum amylase in the presence of a common duct stone do not always mean that pancreatitis is present. Finally, some individuals produce an abnormal amylase molecule, a condition known as macroamylasemia, which causes persistently elevated amylase levels without evidence of disease. When macroamylasemia is suspected, one can ask the laboratory to send serum to a special laboratory for analysis of the type of amylase responsible.

INDEX

Note: Page numbers followed by *f* indicate figures; those followed by *t* indicate tables.